T0384934

"Dr Trudy Stewart has done it again: written a highly accessible, comprehensive and practical book aimed at newly qualified and therapists starting to specialise in stammering. I would argue that 100 Navigation Points is also useful for experienced speech and language therapists looking to keep up-to-date with the latest thinking on therapy approaches for young people and adults who stammer.

Navigating Adult Stammering has a pleasing logical structure, starting (quite rightly) with the person who stammers, moving onto the therapist and the relationship between the two, before describing a range of therapy approaches. In this way the reader gains an overview of the different options available. The book is peppered with useful example of real people Trudy has worked with over the years and their stammering therapy journeys, bringing to life the therapy process. In this way Trudy generously shares her skills and knowledge and is not afraid to describe when she has not always got things right and what she learnt from those experiences. In line with this desire to share learning from others, she includes comments from practising therapists reflecting on what they wish they had known at the start of their work with dysfluent clients.

Another useful feature occurring throughout the book is the way Trudy highlights commonly occurring difficulties/challenges and possible solutions when describing particular ways of working. In this way Trudy skilfully anticipates the questions often posed by therapists new to the stammering field: 'what do I do if this happens?'. Moreover, she signposts the reader to a list of useful resources at the end of every section.

The two sections which I believe deserve particular mention focus on psychological approaches and the stammer more proudly movement, the former for the way it brings so many different psychological approaches together in one place, the latter for its inclusive and reflective content. For any therapist working in stammering, whether new to the area or experienced, it is incredibly helpful to become more knowledgeable about the ways a client can be supported psychologically and how we as therapists are often the best people to carry out this role.

With regards to the Stammer more proudly section. I was deeply impressed by the way Trudy describes this relatively new way of considering stammering through the lens of the social model of disability. She takes into account ground-breaking work in this area as well as seeking individual views of people who stammer. She does not shy away from reflecting on the potentially uncomfortable questions the stammer more proudly movement pose for us as therapists, and how her own thinking and practice has changed.

In summary, Trudy proves herself once again to be the ultimate clinician's clinician. Drawing upon her decades of working with people who stammer, she offers through this book an invaluable overview and insight into how we as therapists can best empower our clients who stammer."

Rachel Everard, Speech Therapy, City Lit., London

"Recently, the publishing market has come with more and more increasingly valuable publications on stammering. Trudy Stewart's book, although intended for newly qualified speech-language therapists and those just starting to specialize in stammering, will – without a doubt – be enthusiastically received by experienced fluency experts as well. This publication covers all the essential topics related to the stammering intervention. Attentive readers are granted access to both – the primary theoretical content and the details on stammering therapy practice. The publication also discusses the psychological approaches used in stammering. Furthermore, the author explains complex topics, e.g., relapse in stammering therapy. The book is written clearly and reader-friendly while integrating updated knowledge with the author's rich clinical experience. From the very beginning, the reader will confront a holistic and humanistic approach to stammering and people who stammer. This book promotes stammering therapy based on trust, acceptance, and partner cooperation between the speech-language therapist and the clients along with their families and community.

The uniqueness of this book is that it was written by a wise, extraordinarily experienced, and modest professional who emphasizes building a partner relationship from the first moments of contact with the client. The author shows how important it is to become an attentive therapist who can listen to the clients – learn from them and with them. It should be appreciated how open and ready the author is to share her own thoughts, be authentic and sincere in contact with the client. Her eagerness as an SLT to reveal her imperfections is laudable. Her understanding and acceptance toward the stammering phenomenon and individuals who stammer can model her readers. Above all, the commentaries by the experienced clinicians, including the author herself, wishing that they had attained this knowledge when they were newly qualified clinicians have added vital wisdom. These comments are a treasure trove and contain important lessons for any clinician.

I cannot wait for this book to be available in the bookstores. As a professor, I can imagine how meaningful it will be for speech-language therapy students to familiarize themselves with its content. I wish I had had the opportunity to read this book when I took my first steps in stammering therapy."

Professor Katarzyna Węsierska, University of Silesia in Katowice, Poland, European Fluency Specialist & ECSF coach, International Cluttering Association Secretary

"Despite stammering being a core part of Speech and Language Therapy training, the first steps into working with clients who stammer can be daunting. I well remember the anxiety before stepping into the waiting room to greet my first adult client who stammered. What if they ask me something I couldn't answer? Am I up to the job of this 'specialist' area? And, worst of all, what if my lack of experience makes their situation worse? In this book, Dr Trudy Stewart eases the transition into the world of working with adults who stammer by acknowledging these worries and providing clear and sensible steps forward.

Dr Stewart has long been a leading voice in the field of stammering. Her background of clinical work, leadership, research and teaching all have a common thread of 'client-centeredness' woven through them. The same is true from this book. Through these navigational points she provides a road map for working with adults who stammer, but with the reassurance that the final destination isn't ours to know. The client will set the destination and choose the mode of travel. Our job is to help plan the route and make appropriate stop offs at key places.

Through a clearly laid out and accessibly written series of chapters we are guided through this journey; starting with first principals about stammering and challenging the potential preconceptions that newer clinicians may have about their role and purpose when working with adults who stammer, moving through initial meetings and case histories and into the range of therapy and support options we may employ. To do this she draws on well-established ways of working and also introduces newer ideas (e.g., stammer more proudly) with equal weighting to the old. She shares what has worked from personal and shared experiences, as well as discussing what the academic literature has to say on the subject, suggesting stop off points along the way by sign posting resources or further reading for those who wish to delve deeper. Throughout the book Dr Stewart provides a neutral discussion about the range of approaches to working with stammering, placing herself firmly in the midpoint, not pushing a particular approach on the client, but being there to explore options and find what works for them. Each chapter is broken down into short bite sized points to consider along the journey. This allows the reader to dip in and out of the book, using the book as a reference guide and checking in throughout working with the client.

I heartily recommend this book to clinicians taking their first steps into the world of stammering. I'm certain that had this been available to me as a new clinician I would have had a well thumbed copy in the top drawer of my desk at all times. And who knows, I may still do so. Whilst reading this book I couldn't help but reflect on the clients that I'm currently working with, checking in that I had spent enough time at each stage of the journey, making sure that I hadn't missed or over looked part of the process. After all, even experienced travellers need a map sometimes."

Ben Bolton-Grant, Course Director, MSc Speech and Language Therapy, Speech and Language Sciences, Leeds Beckett University

"I never thought I'd say this about a textbook but '100 Navigational Points: Dysfluency' is a great read! The book is filled with an extensive variety of information and approaches which is not only detailed, but clear and comprehensive. From a Speech and Language Therapist (SLT) student's perspective (having not learnt about stammering yet), the book gave me a deep insight into dysfluency and most importantly, individuals who stammer.

Trudy truthfully reflects on her personal growth as a therapist and emphasises the positivity in inexperience; showing your uncertainty and vulnerability is an influential approach when working with a client. I can only imagine how useful this book will be to a therapist who is feeling inexperienced in a role where they are new to stammering. The advice felt relatable and reassuring, whilst reminding me that we, as therapists, should always aspire to self-improve. What traits can I develop further? What can I do now that I wasn't doing before?

The use of hypothetical situations, real-life case examples and analogies helps evoke a profound sense of empathy and understanding from the reader - making the book distinct in contrast to other textbooks. By the end of the book, I felt I had a well-rounded, holistic view of the person who stammers and the various therapy approaches. The use of critical evaluation in the book on perspectives such as the medical and social models of disability also allows the reader to challenge the generalizations and stereotypes associated with stammering.

This book is invaluable to a therapist new to stammering, as Trudy talks about knowledge that she wishes she had known at the start of her role. I really recommend this book, whether it is utilised to update therapists on new research or as a starting out 'go to' resource. I will certainly take forward many of the book's approaches and advice into my future as a SLT."

Isobel Hart, Student Speech & Language Therapist

"Dr. Trudy Stewart has composed a true gift for both Speech and Language Therapists (SLTs) working in the field of Stammering, as well as clients seen by therapists who read this book. I would go as far to say that this brilliantly structured book is a Stammering Therapy Bible for SLTs. Dr. Stewart's wealth of knowledge and experience is admirable, and she has created a practical, applicable, and generalisable guide for SLTs. This book is extremely comprehensive whilst remaining concise and easy to read and navigate, and is essential reading for SLTs in this field. It will support therapists to be truly person-centred, use evidence-based practise, and empower and promote advocacy for a person with a stammer. The incorporation of advice regarding how to be a good therapist and build an appropriate, strong, therapeutic relationship is invaluable. For newly qualified therapists or those starting out in this area, the many therapeutic methods in this field can often feel overwhelming and daunting; however, this book consolidates the extensive volume of research and therapy approaches available into an organised filing cabinet. The anecdotal examples, structure and diagrams make this book highly accessible and enable a therapist to apply their knowledge from this book to their practise. This book is also a fantastic resource for further reading, as Dr. Stewart provides references and recommendations regarding where to find further information on specific areas- essentially, doing all the legwork and saving many hours of research for the reader. Furthermore, this book is highly relevant to current times in terms of considering and exploring newer approaches such as telehealth, the social model to health, the importance of psychological approaches such as mindfulness, and stammering pride. I am truly grateful for Dr. Stewart's ability to create such an enjoyable, comprehensive, and accessible book for which I would like to thank her on behalf of all SLTs with an interest in this area."

Ashleigh Wolinsky, Speech and Language Therapist, Gesher School

"It's far too common to see a great divide in the world of stuttering. The divide between the top of the iceberg and the bottom of the iceberg, between professionals and people who stutter, between the push to change and the need to accept, between the individual journey and the broader movements.

This book weaves it together - presenting a broader range of perspective and experiences. The reader of this book will be smarter about stuttering in general.

And more importantly and far more rare, the reader will understand more of the inside story."

Uri Schneider, MA CCC-SLP, Director, Schneider Speech Faculty, University of California Riverside School of Medicine

NAVIGATING ADULT STAMMERING

This book, the first in an exciting new series, provides speech and language therapy students and newly qualified and beginning stammering specialists with 100 key points that will help form a strong foundation for their work supporting adults and teenagers who stammer.

Composed of practical, relevant and useful advice from an experienced clinician, chapters break advice down into sections which include information about the therapeutic relationship, therapeutic approaches and signposts to further resources. Throughout the book, comments from stammering specialists describe what they wish they had known at the start of their careers.

This book:

- Puts the person who stammers at the heart of therapy, following the clinical choices they might make
- Is written in an accessible style, designed to be dipped in and out of as required
- Draws on the experience of therapists working with those who stammer

Full of advice and guidance to support effective practice, this is an essential resource for anybody new to this client group.

Trudy Stewart is a retired consultant speech and language therapist. She studied in universities in Glasgow, Michigan State (USA) and Leeds. She worked in the UK with children and adults who stammer for nearly 40 years. Her last role was clinical lead of the Stammering Support Centre in Leeds. Trudy has taught undergraduate, graduate and specialist courses for clinicians in the UK, Europe and Sri Lanka, including on the European Clinical Specialisation in Fluency Disorders (ECSF) course. She has carried out research while a clinician, presented her work at international conferences and written several texts on stammering. She recently co-wrote and directed a play about stammering called 'Unspoken.'

NAVIGATING ADULT STAMMERING

100 POINTS FOR SPEECH AND LANGUAGE THERAPISTS

Trudy Stewart

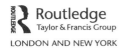

LONDON AND NEW YORK

Cover image: © Getty Images

First published 2022
by Routledge
4 Park Square, Milton Park, Abingdon, Oxon OX14 4RN

and by Routledge
605 Third Avenue, New York, NY 10158

Routledge is an imprint of the Taylor & Francis Group, an informa business

© 2022 Trudy Stewart

British Library Cataloguing-in-Publication Data
A catalogue record for this book is available from the British Library

Library of Congress Cataloging-in-Publication Data
Names: Stewart, Trudy, author.
Title: Navigating adult stammering : 100 points for speech and language therapists / Trudy Stewart.
Description: Milton Park, Abingdon, Oxon ; New York, NY : Routledge, 2022. | Series: Navigating speech and language therapy Includes bibliographical references and index.
Identifiers: LCCN 2021056482 (print) | LCCN 2021056483 (ebook) | ISBN 9781032012544 (hardback) | ISBN 9781032012520 (paperback) | ISBN 9781003177890 (ebook)
Subjects: LCSH: Stuttering—Treatment. | Speech therapy.
Classification: LCC RC424 .S73 2022 (print) | LCC RC424 (ebook) | DDC 616.85/54—dc23/eng/20211220
LC record available at https://lccn.loc.gov/2021056482
LC ebook record available at https://lccn.loc.gov/2021056483

ISBN: 978-1-032-01254-4 (hbk)
ISBN: 978-1-032-01252-0 (pbk)
ISBN: 978-1-003-17789-0 (ebk)

DOI: 10.4324/9781003177890

Typeset in Aldus
by Apex CoVantage, LLC

Access the companion website: www.routledge.com/9781032012520

To all the speech and language therapists and students I have worked alongside, taught and supervised. I have benefitted professionally and personally from your kindness, empathy, good nature, conscientiousness, hard work and humour.

CONTENTS

ACKNOWLEDGEMENTS

This book has been guided and influenced by many colleagues and friends whose various roles I wish to acknowledge here.

First, to my academic friends in the United Kingdom and abroad, in particular Scott Yaruss, Ben Bolton-Grant, Kurt Eggers and Joseph Agius. I am grateful for their guidance on the current status of undergraduate training, which helped me understand what the readership might require of a beginning text on stammering.

Second, thanks to those who espouse the 'stammer more proudly' viewpoint for their conversations and challenges, particularly Katy Bailey, Patrick Campbell, my SLT friend Kath Bond, Kirsten Howell at Stamma and members of the Doncaster self-help group.

I am also grateful to those who shared their answers to the question: 'What do you wish you had known at the start of specialising in stammering?' Their openness and willingness to be vulnerable has been important in guiding the tone of the book.

Thank you to my reviewers, Rachel, Kat, Ben, Uri, Ashley and Isobel, for their very kind and generous endorsements of the book. As a writer, I always wait with some trepidation for the return of reviews. It represents the first time the book has been sent out into the world, and I am never sure if it should be let out on its own at that stage. Getting such wonderful feedback assures me that it is ready to stand on its own bookshelf!

Finally, thank you to my friend Juliette Gregory for her reading of the early drafts and her unending encouragement and positivity. We can now meet for coffee without having to discuss the implications of stammering theory and practice!

And, of course, my wonderful Mark, who in these days of writing has been a constant source of cups of tea/coffee, patience and support. He is my best critic and proofreader and has the ability to make me laugh at myself if it all gets too much.

Thank you all.

INTRODUCTION

In writing this book, I am recalling a time when I was a newly qualified speech and language therapist (SLT). I graduated from Glasgow University and started working at Leeds General Infirmary, where I had enjoyed a final-year clinical placement. The job was a generalist post, and, as such, I was expected to see a variety of children and adults who had usually been referred by their doctor or another medical practitioner. Having no experience other than my student placements, I relied on my undergraduate knowledge, the few clinical competencies I had acquired and, on occasion, the help of other more experienced therapists who worked in the same department.

At that time, it felt like a huge leap to move from a situation where my planning, preparation and delivery of therapy had been monitored and supervised by a senior clinician to one of working totally autonomously. Hopefully that scenario is less likely to occur these days. I clearly remember at different times lacking certainty and confidence and feeling I had only a few tools at my disposal.

I was always nervous when meeting a client for the first time. However, my anxiety was at its highest when the individual presented with a speech or language problem which I had not previously encountered on placement. Thus, there were many sessions in the early months of my career when I imagine I was more ill at ease than the person in front of me.

I vividly recall one situation when a 60-year-old gentleman, who had had a laryngectomy operation, came for a session. At that time, post-laryngectomy voice was created using oesophageal air, a method of voice production I had never seen taught, nor could I mimic myself. I prepared for the session by reading all the texts I could find and re-reading my undergraduate notes.

DOI: 10.4324/9781003177890-1   1

The initial session went well; the man was personable and full of good humour. I wonder now if he could see my inexperience and worked hard to put me at ease. The story has a happy ending in that he learnt to use an excellent oesophageal voice and went on to give talks about his surgery and living without a larynx to pre-operative individuals and local groups. The point I take away from this encounter is that I had little or no experience on which to base my management of this situation, but despite that, the outcome was positive. And why was that? It was not fundamentally due to any knowledge I imparted to him from the textbooks or notes, nor the bluff and bluster of my knowledge-sharing techniques or explanations. More likely, it was the client's wonderful positivity, motivation and good nature; the relationship we shared; and the mutual sense of learning and problem solving that arose from the sessions.

These memories and reflections are at the forefront of my mind when I write this textbook. I write about what I wish I had known in those early forays into a career in speech and language therapy. I am writing what a more experienced clinician would tell my younger self, and I hope that from reading those words, a less accomplished reader will be empowered to be the best therapist they can be.

(I have not relied on my own wisdom but requested contributions from therapists currently embarking on a career as specialists in stammering, including therapists who had recently graduated from the European Clinical Specialization in Fluency Disorders [ECSF]. I asked them what they wished they had been told as newly qualified clinicians, and some of their remarks, which were generously provided, are included as small 'cameos' outside the main text.)

The text is organised into a number of sections, with multiple navigation points included in each. The sections mark a hypothetical clinical journey which will always start and end with the person who stammers (PWS). The clinician and her relationship with the PWS is introduced, and its importance comes second only to that of the client. Beginning sessions are described, with attention given to a number of strategies which I consider generic in the management of stammering. The sections which follow then present some therapy options which can be offered to the PWS and from which a jointly negotiated management plan will emerge. Relapse management is given a separate section rather than being included in the general section on therapy. This reflects the importance I believe it has in the attainment of the person's long-term therapy objectives. The final section, on support networks, reflects the holistic approach that must be used when working with a PWS. The involvement of significant others (SOs) in his life will ensure that the changes he seeks to make in therapy are integrated into the whole of his life and not limited to the clinic room.

I have tried to use an accessible style throughout the book. The use of the abbreviation PWS for a person who stammers was chosen to reflect that each person who stammers is an individual in his own right and not an unidentified 'stammerer'. I have used 'he' to refer to each person who stammers and 'she' to refer to a therapist. This reflects the majority of males and females in each group, but I am aware that this is not an accurate representation. My apologies to females who stammer and male SLTs who may feel unrepresented and excluded. This was not my intention.

Finally, after 40 years of working in this special field of stammering, writing this text has taught me, yet again, that stammering is incredibly complex. It can be challenging for any therapist, whether one is newly qualified or well experienced and seemingly knowledgeable. There is much to learn and a great deal yet to be discerned. However, clinicians everywhere have access to the best source of knowledge and experience possible; the PWS himself.

Section A

THE PERSON WHO STAMMERS

We start where everyone wishing to understand stammering should begin: by listening and trying to understand the issues from the perspective of the person who knows the most. For a clinician meeting a person who stammers (PWS) in her clinic for the first time, what can she anticipate?

1. GENERIC FEATURES

Are adults who stammer different in some way? Research shows that, as a group, adults who stammer share the same variability of intelligence, sensitivity, anxiety and so on as the general population. Alm (2014) reviewed studies of people who stammered and found that individuals were not 'characterized by constitutional traits of anxiety or similar constructs' (p. 5). As such, a SLT cannot assume that specific issues and/or characteristics will be the same for every client and should approach each PWS as an individual.

2. STATE OF SELF

A client may come to his first session feeling excited and keen to engage with the process. For others, the starting point may be a dark and isolated place, with little or no hope. Stewart and Brosh (1997) describe some clients who were in difficult places when they came for therapy.

It can be quite scary for an SLT lacking in experience to encounter such a person and hear his situation. However, often these are the individuals who do best in therapy; they have the most to gain and can travel the furthest from their first session to amazing outcomes. I would not wish to generalise and say that is true for all, but I do encourage clinicians to start

DOI: 10.4324/9781003177890-2

from a position of hope, as this will rub off onto the PWS. For example, using positive statements regarding affirmation and attainment are helpful: 'You might not be able to see your way through this at the moment, but on our journey together you will find out that you know more, can do more and can achieve more than you think.'

3. STAMMERING FEATURES

There are no typical features of stammering which can be assumed; each PWS has a unique stammering profile which, as we see later in this book, may or may not consist of observable features and may or may not involve psychological responses. An individual can present with multiple overt behaviours and little or no covert (or hidden) issues. Another person will have few if any observable signs of stammering but a multitude of psychological responses to his stammering.

An important study by Tichenor and Yaruss (2019) looked at how adults who stammered identified and experienced stammering. They found that participants viewed stammering as an experience with many facets:

- different emotions (including shame, guilt, worry, anxiety, embarrassment, emotional pain, hopelessness, emotional exhaustion and fear)
- cognitions (including thoughts relating to anticipation, identity, sense of self and self-esteem)
- behaviours (including overt features – prolongations, repetitions and blocks – and covert features – including choosing not to speak, removing themselves from a situation, substituting feared sounds or words or using other methods to hide or avoid detection by conversation partners)
- limitations (including not being able to say what they want to say in a conversation, difficulties forming social relationships, being denied or limited in larger life opportunities such as career or education)
- negative consequences.

"To adults who stutter, the term stuttering signifies a constellation of experiences beyond the observable speech disfluency behaviors that are typically defined as stuttering by listeners. Participants reported that the moment of stuttering often begins with a sensation of anticipation, feeling stuck, or losing control. This sensation may lead speakers to react in various ways, including affective, behavioral, and cognitive reactions that can become deeply ingrained as people deal with difficulties in saying what they want to say. These reactions can be associated with adverse impact on people's lives. This interrelated chain of events can be exacerbated by outside environmental factors, such as the reactions of listeners."

(Tichenor & Yaruss 2019, p. 4356)

Observable stammering features reported generally in the literature and observed in a clinical setting include:

- repetitions; often of plosive consonants, but this can be of other sounds
- prolongations, of both consonants and vowels
- blocks/silent prolongations, that is, stopping of the production of a sound. This can be at the laryngeal or articulatory level
- hard articulatory attack
- breathing disruptions
- other verbal issues e.g. added extras; fillers, such as ers, ums
- tension in face, larynx, diaphragm or other parts of the body e.g. legs, arms, hands
- physical concomitant movements or secondary body movements e.g. hand rubbing, foot tapping
- eye contact; e.g. lack of eye contact, fixed eye gaze, flickering eye movements
- disruptions in speech rate; e.g. too fast, too slow or inconsistent rate
- other non-verbal behaviours; e.g. those involving facial expression, posture.

Covert and psychological responses to stammering include:

- avoidance: sound, word, speech, situation, feeling, relationship self-role (Sheehan 1970) and intention to behave (Stewart 2012)
- emotional responses before, during and after stammering
- unhelpful thoughts; criticisms, negativity, guilt, suicidal thoughts
- unhelpful feelings; self-degradation, depression, shame, lack of self-respect, loss of pride
- unhelpful behaviours; neglect, isolation
- anxiety; generalised and/or specific (e.g. related to certain situations; particular people).

A comprehensive discussion of both observable features and covert and psychological responses can be found in Turnbull and Stewart (2017).

4. REASONS FOR WANTING THERAPY

In preparing to meet a client for the first time, a clinician must have a completely open mind regarding the issues which concern the person and his motivations for seeking therapy. They may be different from anything that has been written by the referring agency. In my experience, the original reasons a PWS decides to come for therapy are wide ranging, including wanting to say wedding vows, being able to read a bedtime story to a child, trying to understand stammering and particular psychological reactions to it. These reasons may or may not be related to a desire to increase fluent speech.

5. KNOWLEDGE ABOUT STAMMERING

A PWS often has little or no knowledge of what stammering is, the theories pertaining to it, relevant research or treatment options available. A person may have avoided references to stammering and shied away from reading articles in newspapers or features in popular magazines about others who stammer or so-called miracle 'cures' that have been found. This is often part of his coping strategies: not thinking about stammering or engaging with anything to do with it. Another individual, however, will have read widely and looked at numerous internet sites. Consequently, he has lots of questions, which could be challenging to a newly qualified therapist who is perhaps not as well versed in online resources at this stage in her career. If such a situation occurs, it is advisable for the SLT to read the literature alongside the person and talk about it together with him, using the material as a discussion point and a basis for being open about stammering.

6. UNDERSTANDING OF STAMMERING

A PWS comes to his own understanding of stammering based on a range of factors. These include his personality, the way he construes and thinks about things generally, his cultural background, previous experiences with other PWSs and other people's reactions to his stammer (i.e. family members, teachers and other significant people in his life). Once again, it is important for the therapist not to assume that the person has the same understanding of stammering as she does, nor a desire for fluency and/or an intolerance of dysfluency.

7. UNDERSTANDING OF THERAPY

A few adults who present for therapy have no previous experiences of therapy. However, many individuals come into the clinic room carrying with them memories of therapy sessions as a child. These may have been quite pleasant encounters with the

> I wish I had known how to learn more about the client's previous therapy experiences. Now I know that understanding therapy that has gone before helps us (the SLT) to better understand how to orientate our management.
> Francesca del Gado (Personal Communication 2021)

'speech lady', perhaps remembered for having great toys and playing fun games. However, in some instances, the encounters are recalled with negativity. One person talked about her feelings of failure as she struggled to use the speech techniques anywhere but the clinic room, a problem encountered by many. These feelings of failure, negativity, frustration and so on will impact on the PWS in an adult therapy context. His assumptions of what will happen in therapy and the emotional responses he expects can be barriers to the therapy process.

It is therefore important that the clinician explore and enable the person to give voice to his concerns and worries based on any past encounters. She can then address his anxieties and set the foundations for a new and different experience.

8. OUTCOMES

A crucial topic for discussion in early therapy sessions, if not in the first meeting, is to establish what the PWS hopes to achieve from therapy. An

> Don't project your own assumptions about stuttering onto the client's life.
> Jo Van der Sypt (Personal Communication 2021)

individual's goals can be simple and relate to a specific situation (e.g. using the telephone at work, ordering lunch fluently in a sandwich shop) or may be more complex (e.g. reducing feelings of isolation, managing negative reactions to stammering in himself and others). An SLT should not assume that every PWS strives to speak fluently and that her role is therefore to teach him techniques relating to speech production which enable that to happen. As we will see in the therapy section, there are many management options open to a PWS, and it is one of the therapist's initial tasks to ensure the individual is aware of the choices available to him. Given the current growing popularity of the social model of disability, (Hunt 1966; Oliver 1990) one choice among many presented to a PWS should be the development of acceptance of stammering, with openness and education of others. (See **Section E, Point 45.**)

Once the desired outcomes for a person are established, they will influence the subsequent assessment and development of a holistic management programme.

9. STAGES OF CHANGE

In order to determine where therapy should start, a clinician needs to know where the person is in his process of change. In trying to understand the process of change, including a person's readiness to engage, Prochaska and DiClemente developed a model based on six stages of change.

It is very helpful to identify these recognised stages with a PWS, as they can guide the management of therapy. The stages of change model helps a therapist to identify and advise an individual on his readiness to change. It also enables her to choose an appropriate strategy to facilitate a person to move forward and into active change. This improves outcomes and efficacy of therapy while acknowledging that relapse or difficulty in maintaining gains is an important learning process and not a failure for either the PWS or the clinician.

> Sometimes people are still just in the "precontemplation phase" of their process and it seems too soon to start therapy. Or sometimes people try therapy because someone else decided it would be good for them. Therefore I would have liked to know when I started that it's okay to be slow in the beginning and take enough time to talk about the goals and reasons why they want to start therapy.
> Monica Rocha (Personal Communication 2021)

The stages of change are outlined in the following paragraphs, accompanied by therapy ideas for each stage. However, reading of the following texts will be useful for a newly qualified practitioner: Stewart in press 2022; Turnbull 2000; Prochaska & DiClemente 1982, 1992; Prochaska et al. 1992; McConnaughy et al. 1983.

i. Precontemplation
    In this stage, a person does not acknowledge that he needs to think, feel or do anything differently. This may be because he is unaware of a problem, denies that a difficulty exists or feels unwilling or unable to change. If an individual comes for therapy while at this stage, it is often because some other person (e.g. a partner, friend, relative) has suggested it.

    Therapy is difficult at this stage, but the following techniques are suggested: empathy, reflective listening, providing choices, the use of paradox (i.e. 'So what will be the result of doing more of what you are currently doing?'), instilling hope and exploring those issues which he sees as barriers to change.

ii. Contemplation. A person in this stage has moved to accept that a problem exists, but he is ambivalent about what to do to solve the situation. He is fearful of both the status quo and the possibility of change in the future.

> 🏮 It would have been useful to know that some people are actually not really open for help. Even though they don't want to stutter they are not willing to change their behaviour and thoughts.
>
> Jo van der Sypt (Personal Communication 2021)

Therapy strategies for this stage are:

a. conversations which allow the client to understand his ambivalence and move him to making a decision and

b. self-evaluation techniques (that is, those which help him look at the implications of change, to weigh up the pros and cons of both staying the same and of change).

iii. Preparation. This is a stage during which there is an intention to change and indeed some attempt to change. It may be short in duration, and it is important that the therapist and PWS recognise the readiness and capitalise upon it. If missed, the individual may move back into the previous stages.

Therapy strategies here are:

a. raising the client's awareness about how he feels and thinks about himself in relation to the problem and

b. helping him choose and commit to an act of change by making a decision or a resolution and committing to it.

iv. Action.

In the action stage, there is an awareness of cognitive, emotional and/or behaviour change. Such changes may be noticed by a clinician or a person's 'significant other' or may only be noticed by the individual himself.

The therapist's role in this stage is to present choices or alternatives from which the PWS can choose to experiment. It is important that this experimentation continue for as long as possible, as it helps to maintain the change. The SLT will play a role in supporting and acknowledging the difficulties as these experiments proceed.

Therapy strategies include:
a. desensitisation, relaxation and assertiveness training to 'toughen' a PWS to adverse reactions and negative thoughts or emotions;
b. increased openness about stammering and enlisting others to act as triggers or reminders to a person to act in the way he has chosen; and
c. building in rewards for times when the changes are achieved.

v. Maintenance.

The maintenance stage prepares a person for times when it is difficult to sustain the gains that have been made. At this point, he develops strategies which keep his change(s) in place.

Therapy strategies: The client should be encouraged to collect ideas or tools from the beginning of his therapy to enable him to create and develop a personal tool box of strategies for this maintenance stage. (For more detailed description of tool boxes and their development and an example of a completed tool box, see **Section J, Point 92**, and the maintenance chapter in Turnbull & Stewart 2017.)

vi. Termination.

I think it is useful to think about termination in the context of when a person is moving away from therapy. In my experience, a client often knows when he is ready and will suggest this to his therapist in a variety of ways, for example, mentioning he has a new hobby or has joined a new social group, thus indicating he has new priorities and less time for therapy and is moving on in his life.

REFERENCES

Alm, P.A. (2014). Stuttering in relation to anxiety, temperament and personality: Review and analysis with focus on causality. *Journal of Fluency Disorders*, 40, 5–21.

Hunt, P. (1966). *Stigma: The Experience of Disability*. London: Geoffrey Chapman.

McConnaughy, E.A., Prochaska, J.O. & Velicer, W.F. (1983). Stages of change in psychotherapy: Measurement and sample profiles. *Psychotherapy: Theory, Research & Practice*, 20, 368–375.

Oliver, M. (1990). *The Politics of Disablement*. London: Macmillan Publishers Limited.

Prochaska, J.O. & DiClemente, C.C. (1982). Transtheoretical therapy: Toward a more integrative model of change. *Psychotherapy Theory Research & Practice*, 20, 161–173.

Prochaska, J.O. & DiClemente, C.C. (1992). Stages of change in the modification of problem behaviors. In M. Herson, R.M. Eisler & P.M. Miller (eds.), *Progress in Behavior Modification*, vol. 28. Il: Sycamore.

Prochaska, J.O., DiClemente, C.C. & Norcross, J.C. (1992). In search of how people change: Applications to addictive behaviors. *American Psychologist*, 47, 1102–1114.

Sheehan, J.G. (1970). *Stuttering: Research and Therapy*. New York: Harper & Row.

Stewart, T. (2012). Avoidance in adults who stutter: A review and clinical discussion. *Polish Forum Logopedyczne*, 20, 20–29.

Stewart, T. (In press, proposed publication date 2022). The narrative of personal change. In K. Eggers & M. Leahy (eds.), *Case Reports in Stuttering and Cluttering*. London: Routledge, Taylor & Francis Group.

Stewart, T. & Brosh, H. (1997). The use of drawing in the management of adults who stammer. *Journal of Fluency Disorders*, 22, 1, 35–50.

Tichenor, S.E. & Yaruss, J.S. (2019). Stuttering as defined by adults who stutter. *Journal of Speech, Language & Hearing Research*, 62, 12, 4356–4369.

Turnbull, J. (2000). The transtheoretical model of change: Examples from stammering. *Counselling Psychology Quarterly*, 31, 1, 13–21.

Turnbull, J. & Stewart, T. (2017). *The Dysfluency Resource Book*, 2nd edition. London: Routledge.

OTHER RESOURCES

Cheasman, C., Everard, R. & Simpson, S. (2013). *Stammering from the Inside: New Perspectives on Working with Young People and Adults*. Havant: J.R. Press.

Section B

THE THERAPIST

 ## 10. WHO AM I TO BE?

An inexperienced clinician might wonder 'Who am I to be?' in an interaction with a PWS or indeed any client coming to her clinic. The answer is simple: genuinely yourself. When working as a clinical supervisor, I remember a senior academic visiting a second-year student SLT who was on placement with me. The visiting clinician was critical of the student for her interactions with the client. She told the trainee that she should 'not be herself but act the role of a therapist'. This angered and confused me and continues to reverberate, as it runs counter to my own understandings of how to interact with a client. It is my belief one should fundamentally be oneself with a person while being aware of the impact any non-verbal signals, communication style and other behaviours might have. Being true to oneself is inherently therapeutic: in Rogerian terms, being genuine.

For my clinical practice, this has meant, on occasions, I have actively challenged and chastised individuals; laughed and cried with PWS and families; and disclosed things about myself when it was safe, relevant and therapeutic for the client. Being this way also means a clinician takes off the protection that playing a role other than herself might give. I am sure this advice could be challenging for a newly qualified therapist, but being oneself is a certain way to build a genuine relationship with a client, which is fundamental to effective therapy.

11. WHAT WOULD A PERSON WHO STAMMERS VALUE FROM HIS CLINICIAN?

There are a number of studies which investigate the various values that adult clients believe are desirable in an SLT.

 DOI: 10.4324/9781003177890-3

Haynes and Oratio (1978) found that skilful interpersonal proficiency in a therapist was considered essential, with empathic genuineness (i.e. listening in a careful and

> At the start I thought I was supposed to have answers. Now I think it is better not to know and to care.
> Phil Schneider (Personal Communication 2021)

accepting way), a sense of humour and not playing a false role all thought to be vital. Crane and Cooper (1983) also state that assertiveness, flexibility and confidence were rated as crucial elements of clinical effectiveness. Similarly, Fourie (2009) reported on the nature of being therapeutic as described by adult clients with acquired communication and swallowing disorders. The factors included being understanding, erudite, inspiring, confident, soothing, practical and empowering.

12. THE CLINICIAN'S JOURNEY

It is important to acknowledge that a clinician is on a journey in the same way her clients are. She is learning about therapy, how to be a therapist and the different forms of stammering with each person that comes to see her. She will have times on that road when she feels less confident than others, and it is essential to recognise those challenging times alongside the other occasions when things go amazingly well. Acknowledging openly to a PWS that she does not know will be an excellent way of empowering him and validating his role as expert in the therapeutic process.

13. BEING PERSON CENTRED

Much is written about the importance of a therapist using this approach (Rogers 1967), but what does it equate to in practice? It means if I am bored or irritated by a PWS, I am not being person centred. If I am thinking my own thoughts, such as, 'What am I going to have for lunch?', or 'Will I be able to finish that report before going home?', I am not being person centred. If a therapist *is* being person centred, then the most important person in the room is the PWS. She is completely focused on him, and all her personal concerns have been placed at the back of her mind, out of reach. She is aware of his concerns; whether he needs a drink of water, a pen and paper, a tissue or a more comfortable seat. She concentrates on what the individual has to say and may jot down on paper some key words or phrases he uses because she wants to remember and use them in future conversations with him.

While this can seem like a therapist sitting back and absorbing, as we will see in the section on the therapeutic relationship, it also involves using and applying all her knowledge and understanding of stammering. So, at points, she will question, raise new pertinent points and propose hypotheses for experimentation and testing out.

 ## 14. LISTENING

The most important skill a therapist has is the ability to listen effectively. In a good therapy session, the client will be talking 80% of the time, which means the clinician will be talking 20% and listening 80%. Active listening involves not just hearing the content of the PWS's narrative but the manner in which it is delivered and, sometimes, what is not being disclosed. When training undergraduates, I suggest listening like a rabbit, that is, with one's whole self, being still, concentrating, even metaphorically sniffing the air! Active listening also involves making subtle responses so when a person says something which might be important to his change process, a word or phrase which needs to be reinforced, underlined or enhanced, then the therapist will draw attention to it by nodding or affirming it in some other way.

Listening is also about creating a space in which the individual has time to talk. Campbell (2020) gives an example of his experience of being given this time by a therapist:

> I once went to a therapy session with stuttering as far as possible from my mind. I had sat some important medical exams and suspected (incorrectly, it turned out) I had failed them. I had a forty minute session booked; I came out two hours later.

We hadn't spoken much at all about my stuttering; instead, my therapist had offered support, comfort and a listening ear at an anxiety provoking time for me. I'm very grateful to this day for that session that boosted my spirits and settled my nerves.

Occasionally, a stutterer will turn up to therapy in a mindset in which they are not able to engage in therapy around their stutter; the session is not lost. You can still listen to the person in front of you and help them a little on their life journey.

(Campbell 2020)

15. ACCEPTANCE AND POSITIVE REGARD

In a conference presentation (Stewart 2005), I once described how a therapist metaphorically holds up a mirror to her client, saying 'Look; this is the great person you are.' While being a witness to his narrative, the SLT reflects back to him his positive qualities and, in so doing, enables the PWS to develop a more nurturing attitude and ultimately to feel better about himself.

Sometimes acceptance may run counter to a clinician's beliefs. She may close down the person's dialogue and move him onto a different topic area because the content is hard for her to manage. A therapist needs to be aware of her own responses to what is being disclosed and seek support where she feels this is required. I once met a client who told me how angry he was with his stammer. There were underlying reasons for this, which were acknowledged in the therapy sessions. One day he told me that his anger had got the better of him, and he had initiated a violent encounter with a young man. As a pacifist at heart, this would have disturbed me had I not been in a clinical setting. However, I accepted his actions, and we sought to make sense of it together and to work out a way to channel and then resolve his anger. (He referred himself for counselling to do this, recognising that it was something he could work on separately from issues with his communication.)

16. EMPATHY

Often rated as the most helpful of counselling skills by clients (Egan 2001), empathy is the way a therapist connects with her client's experience through a number of underlying elements. Brown (2018) suggested five major elements of empathy that can be learned:

i.   to see the world as another sees it, or perspective taking
ii.   to be nonjudgmental
iii. to understand another person's feelings
iv.   to communicate your understanding of that person's feelings
v.   to practise/develop mindfulness, or pay attention.

With regard to the understanding of the client, Mair (1989), the exceptional Personal Construct psychologist and writer, talked about 'standing under' the person's experience and, like a waterfall, letting it wash over you. He writes in poetic form:

Understanding requires
putting yourself in a position
to be taught by
to learn from
to experience
to be affected and changed
to be humble
to stand under
Not to be aloof
different
superior
separate
high up
out of reach
remote
professionally untouchable
To understand
is to be drenched
and washed and

flowed over by
It is to take the form
of the other
to give your form away
and in yourself to assume
the form of the other
so that you can be
informed thereby
It is to become
a pupil
It is to care enough
to give the other
power

(p. 157)

Thus, a therapist participates in the client's experience from a personal perspective rather than from some objective disconnected viewpoint.

She starts by attending and listening well. Then, during this process, she tries to stand in the person's shoes, accepting the way they fit, and positively reinforces and affirms his thoughts and feelings.

17. USING AFFIRMATIONS

Affirmations are clinician's statements used to underline something the individual has said which contributes to his change process. They also validate success or achievements. Affirmations can be used:

- to mark progress when specific targets have been met ('I know how much work has been involved here, and now your efforts are getting results')
- when difficult disclosures have been made in conversation: (e.g. 'It's great that you have told me about this. Well done')
- where a client has 'blind spots' that is, areas about which he is unaware
- to draw attention to certain skills and abilities he has which would help him move forward (e.g. 'Have you noticed how

you were able to keep eye contact while talking about that very anxious situation? That's quite a change for you. How were you able to do that?').

18. SUMMARISING

In this technique, a therapist draws together two or more of the client's thoughts, feelings or behaviours, and make connections he may not readily see. For example, 'You are trying to "bring out" your stammer with your girlfriend but you fear she is going to "go off" and not have time to listen.' Here, using his words, the therapist has linked an individual difficulty with being open to his pre-emptions about his girlfriend's reactions. It is very important when using summarising to employ the person's own words and phrases where possible. This reinforces the client as the author of his own narrative and the person holding the power and control. (This is an important point when we come to look at the therapeutic relationship.)

19. HUMOUR

This sense of fun and creative use of language has been written about in the context of stammering therapy by Manning (2009) and Agius (2018).

Humour has been found to strengthen rapport, facilitate cooperation, increase the person's coping skills and be an alternative way of seeing situations for a client. Used sensitively, it can provide a useful release of tension when the discussion revolves around difficult issues. Consequently, a therapist should not be afraid of using humour in a session; it helps build the relationship with a PWS, acts to 'lubricate the therapy process' (Agius 2018) and makes her feel better, too!

To find out how to develop the use of humour (as a clinician or of a client), have a look at: the 7 Humor Habit Program in McGhee's book *Humor as Survival Training for a Stressed Out World* (2010).

20. SILENCE

Silence may be quite challenging in an individual session with a person. An inexperienced therapist can feel any silence is her responsibility, perhaps representing some sort of uncertainty, failure or mistake on her part. As a result, she will often jump in with a comment to fill the space in the communication. However, silence is therapeutic. When a clinician has asked a difficult question or made a challenging remark, an individual needs time and space to process his response. When listening like a rabbit (see **point 14**), a therapist can observe the cogs turning for the PWS and should get a sense of when it would be appropriate to speak. In my experience, it is often in these quiet moments that profound meaning can be found; I have seen big pennies drop at such times.

Silence can also be a tool. For example, to challenge a PWS to take responsibility for equal turn taking in the topic being discussed, to encourage him to express his feelings or thoughts and contribute previously unspoken aspects of his story.

It is useful for an inexperienced therapist to build up her tolerance of silence, to get used to just sitting attentively and waiting for the individual to process what is in his head.

In addition, when experimenting with using silence with a person, a clinician can establish what is helpful by asking the individual directly. She can establish when thinking time is required (e.g. 'Is this a point to stop and think about this issue?') and what sort of time he needs (e.g. 'Shall I give you a couple of moments to think about this?'). By asking these overt questions, the silence is negotiated, and as a result, the clinician will be able to better punctuate her communication in a way which is appropriate to her client's needs.

21. REFLECTIVE SKILLS

Two factors which research has shown to differentiate between effective and less effective therapists, according to Wampold (2015), are to:

> "express more professional self-doubt, and engage in more time outside of the actual therapy practicing various therapy skills."

> (p. 273)

First, the expression of doubt is interesting, as some might regard this as uncertainty and a lack of confidence. However, in expressing this hesitancy, the clinician has already looked at her own practice with a critical eye, and such self-reflection is to be encouraged. It is through this mechanism that a therapist will grow and mature in her work.

The second factor of practice can be difficult for a clinician working alone. Nevertheless, talking to colleagues, peer support groups and reading widely should achieve some positive results. Using mindfulness and active listening techniques with friends and family will also potentially benefit all involved and give the SLT valuable skills practice.

Reflection in the moment of clinical interaction is a difficult skill and may need to be developed through the support of regular clinical supervision. The process of supervision allows an SLT to consider her practice 'after the event' and to be challenged and questioned on the interactions between herself and her clients. This reflection can then be used to inform therapeutic work in the future.

22. SPECIFIC SKILLS

Stewart and Leahy (2010) discuss the importance of a therapist being able to engage in evidence-based practice when working with a PWS. In order to accomplish this, they state that SLTs must have a number of skills at their disposal:

- the ability to adopt an hypothesis testing approach
- have access to evidence to assess others' experiences with different treatment approaches
- have well-developed critical evaluation skills in order to appraise the available evidence
- be able to assess the client's circumstances and recommend management options in a way that is meaningful to and motivates the client
- be able to record and reflect on the dynamics of the therapeutic process.

23. LANGUAGE AND MESSAGES TO THE PWS

A non-judgmental, accepting therapeutic stance should be reflected in the language a clinician uses with her client. The way she talks about his speech and the level of fluency or stammering he is experiencing also needs to be non-judgmental. Fluency is not good or bad; stammering is not bad or good. So, a therapist will *not* be saying: 'Well done, you said that without stammering' or 'Your stammering is worse today.' Imagine the scenario where the individual decides he wishes to talk more fluently and a 'speak more fluently' approach is agreed on as the course of action. The clinician then praises the development of his fluency or lack of fluency during the sessions. Then, sometime later, the client feels that changing the spontaneity of his talking is too great a price to pay for more fluency, and he wishes to look at other options. Can he go back to this therapist, who has demonstrated in her interaction with him how she values his level of fluency highly, and ask for an alternative approach? How can the therapist change her feedback and now praise open stammering with any credibility?

Instead, the therapist must comment on the specific techniques of a particular approach: the person's openness, his breathing, levels of tension, non-avoidance and so on and always value the content of his utterance over and above the way he speaks.

24. BEING AN AMBASSADOR FOR THE STAMMERING COMMUNITY

Finally, I believe therapists working with adults and children who stammer have a wider role to play, especially those who aspire to be or who are specialists in this field. I think it is incumbent upon us to be ambassadors for the stammering community, playing a part in supporting their activities, promoting stammering charities and affiliated groups, contributing to such event as stammering open days and the

International Stammering Awareness Day (ISAD; Oct 22) and the annual International Stuttering Online Conference. However, clinicians should be careful not to speak for their clients; therapists might be experts in therapy, but they are not the experts in stammering. Individuals who stammer are the experts. (See more on this in **Section H, Stammer More Proudly**.)

Here in the United Kingdom, Action for Stammering Children has built a great repository of videos by 'Stambassadors', people who stammer in a range of jobs, showing that a PWS can be anything he wants to be with a stammer.

REFERENCES

Agius, J. (2018). Shifting perceptions: Using creativity and humor in fluency intervention. *Forum Logopedyczne*, 26, 49–61.

Brown, B. (2018). *Dare to Lead*. London: Penguin Random House.

Campbell, P. (2020). *How to Be a Stuttering Therapist*. Stuttering Therapy Resources. www.stutteringtherapyresources.com/blogs/blog/how-to-be-a-stuttering-therapist [Accessed 8 March 2021].

Crane, S.L. & Cooper, E.B. (1983). Speech-language clinician personality variables and clinical effectiveness. *Journal of Speech & Hearing Disorders*, 48, 2, 140–145.

Egan, G. (2001). *The Skilled Helper: A Problem-Management Approach to Helping*. Pacific Grove, CA: Brooks Cole Publishing Co.

Fourie, R.J. (2009). A qualitative study of the therapeutic relationship in speech and language therapy: Perspectives of adults with acquired communication and swallowing disorders. *International Journal of Language & Communication Disorders*, 44, 6, 979–999.

Haynes, W.O. & Oratio, A.R. (1978). A study of clients' perceptions of therapeutic effectiveness. *Journal of Speech & Hearing Disorders*, 43, 1, 21–23.

Mair, M. (1989). *Between Psychology and Psychotherapy: A Poetics of Experience*. London, New York: Routledge.

Manning, W.H. (2009). *Clinical Decision Making in Fluency Disorders*. Canada: Singular Thompson Learning.

McGhee, P. (2010). *Humor as Survival Training for a Stressed Out World: The 7 Humor Habit Program*. Bloomington, IN: AuthorHouse.

Rogers, C.R. (1967). *On Becoming a Person: A Therapist's View of Psychotherapy*. London: Constable & Constable Ltd.

Stewart, T. (2005). *The Artist's Eye*. Keynote presentation at 7th Oxford Dysfluency Conference, St Catherine's College, Oxford.

Stewart, T. & Leahy, M.M. (2010). Uniqueness and individuality in stuttering therapy. In A. Weiss (ed.), *Perspectives on Individual Differences Affecting Therapeutic Change in Communication Disorders*. New York: Psychology Press.

Wampold, B.E. (2015). How important are the common factors in psychotherapy? An update. *World Psychiatry*, 14, 3, 270–277.

Section C

THE THERAPEUTIC RELATIONSHIP

25. THE IMPORTANCE OF THE THERAPEUTIC RELATIONSHIP

Research has repeatedly shown that the key factor in determining the outcome of therapy, regardless of the type of approach being used, is the relationship which is

> A good relationship with the PWS seems half the success of therapy. Take the time to build it.
> Kato Polfliet (Personal Communication 2021)

established between the therapist and client (Van Riper 1975; Shapiro 1999). Emerick (1974) states:

> "After laboring with stutterers for over a decade I am convinced that it is not only what I do that helps the person get better but also how I do it and who I am."
> (pp. 92–93)

That being the case, it is essential that we understand what components make up such a relationship. Rogers (1967) states that the therapist must use personal characteristics of warmth, empathy, genuineness and unconditional positive regard as a means of establishing a connection with the other person.

But what attributes do both the PWS and clinician need to bring into the encounter for the relationship to be deemed effective?

26. RAPPORT

How to start? When working at the Stammering Support Centre in Leeds, I was lucky enough to have the facilities to make refreshments close at hand. At the start of a session, I would offer the client a drink and go and make this for him

DOI: 10.4324/9781003177890-4

and one for myself. This gave him the opportunity to get comfortable and settle into the clinic room and also gave a message of informality that I was keen to establish.

Small talk: At first, the therapist will chat with the person: make introductions, establish how to address each other, talk about his journey, the weather (in true British style!) or anything that pertains to the moment. Walsh (2007) describes how this serves as a bridge into the business of therapy.

Rapport is two way, so the next stage is for the clinician to hand over the reins of the conversation to the client. This can be done by asking him: 'Where would you like to start?' Immediately the person becomes aware of his 'right to contribute' (Bunning 2004, p. 55) and, indeed, to determine what happens. (This will become an important theme in **Point 29** on balance/power; see subsequent section.) This sharing of responsibilities or mutuality (Walsh & Felson Duchan 2011) can come as a surprise to a PWS who has perhaps not had therapy before or who has experience of a more formal programme or directive style. As such, the therapist should take the opportunity to discuss this type of approach openly 'I would like to work with you on whatever is concerning you right now. I'm keen to hear your story and any ideas for change you might have. Then together we can develop a management plan that will be adapted or changed as we go on.'

27. OPENNESS

The effectiveness of the relationship will depend on how open each of the individuals involved are willing to be. The PWS needs to feel ready and willing to tell his story. This includes those parts which perhaps show him in a less favourable light, those which are full of emotion and those which he may not have disclosed to anyone else. (Bailey 1993).

The therapist, on the other hand, must be willing to hear his story. That may be stating the obvious, but it can be difficult to hear an individual talk about scenarios which are obviously challenging for him. It requires the clinician to sit within the pain the PWS is feeling, which can be a gruelling experience.

I am thinking about situations where I have listened to some tough descriptions, such as contemplations of suicide, childhood abuse, despair. It is therapeutic for the person to recount these troubled events, but there can be a cost to the therapist. Hence, as discussed in **Section B: The Therapist**, there is a need for her to seek support through a supervision process to manage her own feelings and any psychological responses which have been stirred up as a result.

28. SELF DISCLOSURE

Sometimes an exchange will bring to mind something from the clinician's own experience which is akin to that which the PWS describes. It is tempting to share this, but one should always perform a 'health check' on the information first. What will sharing this detail do in the context of the present conversation? If the answer relates to showing empathy or normalising the person's experience, then the test is passed. However, if it serves no purpose other than providing information that the therapist thinks is important or that she feels the need to share in that moment, then the health test is failed.

Self-disclosure, when used appropriately, can be 'a powerful therapeutic ally' that can empower a client to change 'through the appreciation of other people's experiences' (Bailey 1993, p. 45). However, excessive self-disclosure 'is as unhelpful to clients as too little' (p. 46). Any details that the therapist shares must not draw the person's attention away from his own situation to that of the clinician's personal experiences. If the PWS then was curious and asked for more information about what the therapist had undergone, then it would be clear that his focus had shifted and the self-disclosure was untherapeutic.

29. THE BALANCE OF POWER AND CONTROL

There is an inherent asymmetry in a therapeutic relationship; the encounter takes place in a space created by the clinician, who has designated the date and time of the meeting. However, the focus of the session is the client and his need for change.

Frequently the way the discourse takes place underlines the control the therapist has. She initiates conversations, usually by asking questions. She often holds a bank of resources and information which the PWS needs to be made aware of. She may make specific requests of the client, such as suggesting experiments he should carry out, ways of thinking or behaving which may be (jointly) evaluated in subsequent meetings. When the therapy approach is direct, then the powerful, dominant lead role is that of the therapist (or teacher), and the client (learner) role is passive (Stewart & Leahy 2010, 2021).

However, I would argue that when working to empower a PWS, greater symmetry in therapy interaction is preferable, if not essential. This can be achieved by frequently:

• asking the person for his opinion. 'I've seen this used in a similar scenario. I wonder what you think. Do you think it would be appropriate for your situation?'
• adopting a stance of curiosity 'I wonder if you did x, what would happen?' 'I'm curious about z, do you think that it is significant?'
• not being certain. 'I'm not sure about that. It might work or it might not. What do you think?'

30. ASK THE PERSON

A fundamental tenet for a therapeutic relationship is based on George Kelly's so-called First Principle; that is, if you do not know what is going on in a person's mind, ask him. I have put this point in capitals for a reason; I have found this a crucial part of my clinical work. In instances when I do not know the answer to a question, when I am unsure of the way forward or what to do next – I have found asking the PWS to be most helpful.

This way of working can be part of an ongoing process of establishing what works and/or what is working. The therapist may enlist the help of the PWS during a session in reflecting and evaluating his therapy. When an SLT wishes to know what aspects of the dialogue are working or how to develop and improve the questions she is asking, she should not be afraid of consulting the PWS, for example, by asking, 'What question might I ask you now which would be most helpful in moving you forward?' Here the clinician is empowering the PWS to co-construct a conversation with her. He is, in effect, telling her what will work. Simultaneously, the clinician can review the information she has been given and use it to inform subsequent interaction and increase the effectiveness of the dialogue.

Asking the person also means as a therapist, I am not claiming to have all or indeed any answers for my client. This is not a denial of a duty of care but an acceptance that what happens is a dual responsibility of the client and his clinician. The SLT is acknowledging the PWS as the expert, which in the context of his difficulties and his life experience, he is. This understanding can be very liberating for both parties.

31. CHOICE

Another important component in an effective alliance is the creation of a context of choice. Here the individual is presented with options from which he selects the one he thinks best fits his need and circumstances. The clinician does not choose; rather she explains carefully and with as much detail as possible what each option consists of, what the pros and cons are and what the possible outcomes might be in her opinion. In this way, therapy becomes experimentation with alternatives, with no right or wrong way to proceed. The PWS does not make mistakes; rather he finds the best option for him through trying out possibilities, and he is always in control.

Also, this choice making doesn't necessarily involve an either-or scenario; it can include both or combinations of alternatives. For example, Leahy and Wright (1995) describe how a family believed that almonds, being mineral and vitamin rich, could help their child stammer less.

The therapist did not dismiss the family's opinion but recommended work on reducing the child's speech rate as another option. Both options were included in an experiment; with the child eating almonds for two days with no speech work, followed by controlling speech rate for two days and no almonds. A review of the alternatives was carried out at the end.

This context of choice is played out at all levels in therapy, from choosing the therapy approach to the mode of delivery, frequency of appointments and the date and time of the next session.

32. FLEXIBILITY/ADAPTABILITY

Research (Owen & Hilsenroth 2014) has found that rigid adherence to a particular protocol causes issues with the therapeutic alliance and increases the client's resistance to therapy. It was concluded that an approach which was more flexible and accommodating had better outcomes. This is surely a strong argument for ditching the formal programmes and their prescriptive manuals in favour of a non-directive approach with client goals at the heart.

Once a PWS is engaged in therapy and has experienced some change, albeit small, he can have a sense of what else is possible. Often a person will then discuss with his therapist other concerns that he has been thinking about that he would like to work on. This is not an unusual occurrence. Rather than being offputting, I always regarded it as a sign that the individual felt at ease with the process and had confidence in the management plan and therapeutic approach. In these instances, it is important to be flexible and accommodate the person's additional goals, assessing the area first and then building targets into the established process.

33. THE RELATIONSHIP WITH THE SIGNIFICANT OTHER (SO)

Significant others (SOs) are people who play an important part in the PWS's life, e.g a spouse, partner, family members, friends and colleagues. Although the clinician will not have a direct relationship with the client's SO, the influence they exert on the person may well have a bearing on his progress in therapy and therefore should not be ignored. To preempt a scenario where a SO acts in opposition to the goals of therapy, it is useful to involve key SOs at the beginning.

More detail on the importance of an alliance with SO(s) and how to collaborate with them can be found in **Section K: Support Networks**.

REFERENCES

Bailey, R. (1993). *Practical Counselling Skills*. Oxon: Winslow Press.

Bunning, K. (2004). *Speech & Language Therapy Interventions: Frameworks and Processes*. London: Whurr.

Emerick, L. (1974). Stuttering therapy: Dimensions of interpersonal sensitivity. In L.L. Emerick & S.B. Hood (eds.), *The Client-Clinician Relationship: Essays on Interpersonal Sensitivity in the Therapeutic Transaction*. Springfield, IL: Charles C. Thomas.

Leahy, M. & Wright, L. (1995). Therapy for stuttering: Facilitating working with people from different ethnic backgrounds. *Proceedings of 1st World Congress on Fluency Disorders*, 2, 355–360.

Owen, J. & Hilsenroth, M.J. (2014). Treatment adherence: The importance of therapist flexibility in relation to therapy outcomes. *Journal of Counselling Psychology*, 61, 280–288.

Rogers, C.R. (1967). *On Becoming a Person: A Therapist's View of Psychotherapy*. London: Constable & Constable Ltd.

Shapiro, D.A. (1999). *Stuttering Intervention: A Collaborative Journey to Fluency Freedom*. Austin, TX: Pro-Ed.

Stewart, T. & Leahy, M. M. (2010). Uniqueness and individuality in stuttering therapy. In A. Weiss (ed.), *Perspectives on Individual Differences Affecting Therapeutic Change in Communication Disorders*. New York: Psychology Press.

Stewart, T. & Leahy, M. M. (2021). The art and practice of being a clinician working with individuals who stammer. In T. Stewart (ed.), *Stammering Resources for Adults & Teenagers: Integrating New Evidence into Clinical Practice*. London: Routledge.

Van Riper, C. (1975). The stutterer's clinician. In J. Eisenson (ed.), *Stuttering, A Second Symposium*. New York: Harper & Row.

Walsh, I.P. (2007). Small talk is "big talk" in clinical discourse. *Topics in Language Disorders*, 27, 1, 24–36.

Walsh, I.P. & Felson Duchan, J. (2011). Product and process depictions of rapport between clients and their speech-language pathologists during clinical interactions. In R. Fourie (ed.), *Therapeutic Processes for Communication Disorders*. Hove: Psychology Press.

Section D

BEGINNING SESSIONS
The narrative, goal setting and assessment

34. FINDING OUT ABOUT THE OTHER

At the start of a therapeutic encounter, a number of processes are at work. First, both parties are getting to know one another. The client is finding out about the therapist, and in the same way, she is finding out about him. Opinions are formed and judgements made. Fundamental questions are being asked, such as: 'Can I work with this person?' and 'Can I trust him/her?'

The PWS is perhaps wanting to know if the therapist is equipped to deal with his issues. He may wish to know about her background and how she understands stammering. He will be interested in how she converses with him; does she use lots of technical language, or does she talk in a way he can understand? Also, he needs to feel he can trust her, that he can tell her his story and that she will value it. He will form an opinion based on how she listens and reacts to his story.

Meanwhile the clinician tries to use the person-centred skills (Rogers 1967) she knows will be of use at this stage: active listening, openness, affirmation, empathy, being non-judgmental and so on. (See **Section C**.)

35. TAKING TIME TO HEAR THE NARRATIVE

In these early meetings, the individual is asked to tell his story. Usually this is done in the first session. It is a big undertaking for the PWS, and it may be that he is able to partially disclose and share only the factual, non-emotive part. Some of the more difficult issues in his narrative will perhaps emerge over time, and the clinician needs to be patient.

 DOI: 10.4324/9781003177890-5

When asking an individual to talk about close, personal details, the therapist must be aware of the cost to the client. She should give him plenty of time and space and be kind. One important thing to do is to give him warning the session is coming to an end. She should indicate that there are ten minutes or so before the meeting closes and help him to ground himself before leaving the clinic room.

I recall a time when an individual had disclosed some very significant and emotionally charged information to me. I looked at the clock and realised there were only a few minutes before we were due to end the session. Looking at him, I saw clearly he was still feeling the impact of the emotions he had bravely shared with me. I told him we would have to end the session shortly and asked what we needed to do to bring him to a place where he was ready to go back into his day. He said he would appreciate talking about some unrelated issues (i.e. football). This we did until he said he felt okay to leave.

This situation taught me to manage the timing of early encounters better, perhaps allowing 10–15 minutes more when possible, working on grounding exercises or to flag the ending of the session earlier to allow the person to manage his emotions and experience before leaving.

36. HOW NOT TO USE THE CASE HISTORY

When I began working, I think I over-used a case history pro forma I had been introduced to as an undergraduate to guide early sessions. The objective was to obtain all the information deemed relevant on the

> Looking back, I would now tell my younger self to put down the case history pro forma, focus on the PWS and allow him to tell his story.
> Trudy Stewart 2021

form, and consequently, the situation frequently turned into a question-and-answer encounter. It is important in this first meeting to let the PWS do the talking, in the manner he thinks appropriate and with the amount of detail he feels comfortable sharing. If a case history pro forma must be completed for administrative or auditing purposes, the clinician can be writing points down occasionally in order to complete the record after the session. This can be explained to the person in a way which values what he is disclosing, such as, 'I'm just going to write down a couple of things while you talk so I don't forget what you have said.' Where the clinician thinks there are other pieces of information which are missing (for example, information on the family history of stammering and/or details of significant others' reactions to his stammer), then these can be asked after the PWS has finished what he believes are the important issues in his narrative.

This approach contributes to the balance of the relationship; the power and/or control of the narrative is shared. The PWS tells his narrative his way, and the therapist does not 'over question' and asks for minimal amounts of additional information.

37. GOAL SETTING

It is crucial in these early sessions to establish what goals the individual wishes to achieve in therapy. One individual may have thought long and hard about what he wants and can clearly state his objectives. In another situation,

> I guess I was more focused on what I knew should be done in therapy more than what the PWS really wanted. That's why I believe I did not always take into co consideration the specific demand of each patient.
> Selma Saad (Personal Communication 2021)

a person may not be sure about the solution to his problem. In both of these scenarios, I would advocate that the clinician outline all of the options which are available to the PWS. She should be open about:

i.   the approaches which could be followed, for example, 'speak more fluently', stammer more easily, psychological interventions and/or 'stammer more proudly' and what each might involve (e.g. anxiety management techniques, openness and avoidance reduction)
ii. the therapy journey, including the possible effect on the client's emotions, the level of control of his speech, the involvement and reactions of significant others

iii. management options, e.g. individual or group therapy, self-help support.

I have always found goal setting one of the most difficult stages of therapy. I often find myself in a dilemma. Having sat with numerous individuals over several decades, I have seen them go through what can be painful processes to get to their goals. Faced with a person at the beginning of his therapy, do I share with him my experience of others and their processes and warn him of what is possibly ahead if he chooses a certain course of action? Or do I withhold that information and allow him to make his own choices with their consequences? For example, for a PWS who thinks that increased fluency will solve the difficulties he is having at work – I want to tell him about his overall communication skills and the unrealistic dream of perfect fluency and suggest we just move to desensitisation! The problem here is that I am thinking I know better than the PWS; I am presuming I know what he really needs. I am adopting the role of expert and undermining the PWS's choice and self-determination. In fact, I cannot shorten his journey by talking about what I have seen other people do or what others have benefitted from. The individual must travel the road himself, making his own discoveries along the way, which may or may not result in a desensitisation process. He will decide, and every person's journey is different.

There is also a debate about what should be offered to a PWS. Approaches come and go, moving in and out of favour as the research progresses and society and cultural mores develop. Is there an argument that the therapy alternatives offered to a person should also vary with these changes? In the context of the currently popular social model of disability (Hunt 1966; Oliver 1990), I had a discussion with a PWS who advocates 'stammer more proudly'. During the conversation, it was suggested that SLTs should not offer a stammer more fluently approach to clients because it was not the ultimate answer to stammering and fed into the attitude that 'stammering was bad, fluency is best'. While I understand this point of view, I believe a speech and language therapy service and their fluency clinicians have a duty of care to offer all or as many options as possible. I do not feel I can refuse to let a PWS experiment in whatever way he feels he needs to at any particular time. In many ways, I see the clinician as the conduit for a PWS to change and reach an understanding about his stammering. This will be different for each individual and change across the course of a life.

> I wish I had known that not all approach treatments work for every adult, and that it is our job to tailor the treatment to the needs of the PWS.
> Selma Saad (Personal Communication 2021)

38. ASSESSMENTS

The World Health Organization (2001) describes the concepts of impairment, activity limitation and participation restrictions as a way of measuring a disorder such as stammering. (This replaced the earlier terms of disability and handicap.) Using this model, the impairment part of stammering can be measured by looking at overt or surface features of stammering, while the remaining components of the model will be assessed by analysis of the covert features (or below the surface of the iceberg) and the consequences of stammering. Changes in these features are generally used as indicators of the success or failure of interventions. Blomgren (2007) wrote:

> "Any holistic assessment of the success of a stuttering treatment should use a multidimensional approach that includes both impairment and participation restrictions/activity limitations."

> (p. 20)

39. FORMAL ASSESSMENTS

The recommended function of formal assessments with a PWS is to enable areas of stammering to be measured. This can be to establish a baseline from which to move away or to monitor change during therapy. The areas which may be assessed are generally those which research has shown to influence the persistence of the occurrence, severity and/or impact of stammering. In a recent paper by Brundage et al. (2021), 12 experts and researchers provided details of the type of data they collect. They identified six core areas they regarded as important in an assessment process. These were:

- stammering-related background information
- speech, language and temperament development (more applicable for younger clients)
- speech fluency and stammering behaviours
- reactions to stammering by the speaker
- reactions to stammering by people in the speaker's environment
- adverse impact caused by stammering.

In **Appendix 1**, a comprehensive list of formal assessments in current use can be found.

40. INFORMAL ASSESSMENTS

The following can be assessed using informal procedures:

- readiness to change. (See **Section A, Point 9, 'Stages of Change'**)
- stammering presentation; through client and/or SOs reports, clinical observation, checklists, using the stammering iceberg to identify observable features of stammering and internal issues (such as thoughts and emotions)
- stammer – the level at which the breakdown occurs in speech production: articulatory, laryngeal or diaphragmatic, carried out through observation and analysis. (See **Section F, Point 52**, 'Targeting Strategies')
- speech naturalness, that is, how common place the person's speech might appear to an ordinary listener
- impact of stammering; the level of disruption stammering causes in a person's life. This can be assessed through discussion and observation

- avoidance; Sheehan (1970) specifies several levels (sounds, words, speech, feelings, situations, relationships, self-role). In addition, Stewart (2012) describes a further level, which she calls 'intention to behave'. (See **Section E, Point 51**, 'Avoidance Reduction')
- unhelpful thoughts and feelings
- beliefs and attitudes about stammering
- self-description (e.g. diary reports, self-characterisation [Kelly 1955] and self-ratings of stammering severity
- degree of acceptance.

However, not all experts agree on these areas, and there is often a lack of standardisation of the assessments in use. Nevertheless, assessments are used frequently and take up many hours of therapy time to gain a 'holistic' view of the PWS.

41. OUTCOME-BASED ASSESSMENTS

I suggest these as an alternative approach. If the clinician has a full understanding of the person's view of his stammering through the narrative and has negotiated clearly the goals of therapy, then the need for a battery of formal assessments is reduced, if not removed. Assessments can be targeted to the areas the individual wishes to change. Why assess an issue the person does not wish therapy to impact? In physiotherapy terms, it would be like assessing arm function when the issue being treated is tendonitis in the client's knee. In stammering therapy, if the PWS wishes to adopt a 'stammer more easily' approach, then there is no need to take fluency measures. Assess the areas which are targets for change in the negotiated outcomes.

Often as a PWS progresses in therapy and he experiences meaningful change with some issues, he begins to see the possibility of change in other spheres. He may want to include these new areas in his goals for therapy. In this scenario, a clinician can temporarily suspend the ongoing clinical work, assess this new area, establish a baseline for change and then continue on with therapy. In this way, the assessment continues to be relevant to the person, the process and his need.

REFERENCES

Blomgren, M. (2007). Stuttering treatment outcomes measurement: Assessing above and below the surface. *Perspectives on Fluency & Fluency Disorders*, 17, 3, 19–23.

Brundage, S.B., Bernstein-Ratner, N., Boyle, M., Eggers, K., Everard, R., Franken, M-C., Kefalianos, E., Marcotte, A.K., Millard, S., Packman, A., Vanryckeghem, M. & Yaruss, J.S. (2021, September). Consensus guidelines for the assessments of individuals who stutter across the lifespan. *American Journal of Speech-Language Pathology, Clinical Focus*, 30, 6, 2379–2393.

Hunt, P. (1966). *Stigma: The Experience of Disability*. London: Geoffrey Chapman.

Kelly, G.A. (1955). *The Psychology of Personal Constructs: Vols 1 and 2*. New York: WW Norton.

Oliver, M. (1990). *The Politics of Disablement*. London: Macmillan Publishers Limited.

Rogers, C.R. (1967). *On Becoming a Person: A Therapists View of Psychotherapy*. London: Constable & Constable Ltd.

Sheehan, J.G. (1970). *Stuttering: Research and Therapy*. New York: Harper & Row.

Stewart, T. (2012). Avoidance in adults who stammer: A review and clinical discussion. *Polish Forum Logopedyczne*, 20, 20–29.

World Health Organization. (2001). *International Classification of Functioning, Disability, and Health: ICF*. Geneva: WHO.

Section E

THERAPY
General points

42. SERVICE DELIVERY

The options for therapy for a PWS are individual (i.e. face to face or programmed online therapy), group therapy or telehealth, which may be individual or in a group. The choice will depend on what the service can offer and client preferences.

The benefits of individual sessions for a PWS are that they:

- are tailor made
- work on a client's specific goals
- have increased flexibility and adaptations to suit the individual.

The advantages of group therapy for a PWS are that it:

- helps to decreased feelings of isolation
- enables the normalisation of stammering
- facilitates desensitisation of stammering by observing and listening to other individuals who stammer
- increases motivation through working alongside others
- provides peer support during the process of change
- allows experimentation with different roles in the group, e.g. being leader, observer, team member
- reduces the dependence on the clinician; she is not seen as the only source of empathy, wisdom and so on
- provides a more real communication environment with interruptions, disagreements, affirmations and validations occurring naturally.

 DOI: 10.4324/9781003177890-6

In addition, the SLT will find it is an efficient and effective way of managing a large caseload and a positive way of learning from other clinicians when the group is run with more than one therapist.

Telehealth is in its early stages of use. However, research to date shows it can be an effective way of delivering therapy (Burgess 2019).

The advantages of telehealth are that it is:

- convenient for the client
- time efficient for client and therapist
- enables a service to be maintained during a global pandemic.

It is, however, dependent on reliable hardware and software, with the online system located in a secure and suitably quiet environment to minimise distractions and interruptions.

43. ASPECTS OF THERAPY COMMON TO ALL APPROACHES: AN OVERVIEW

This section and the points that follow cover the necessary support mechanisms, 'safety nets' and common interventions which a PWS will find useful to consider and/or learn *before* embarking on a therapy approach. They will be discussed in more detail later in this section.

THERAPY		
Support mechanisms		Safety nets
involving SOs		preparing for change
self-help groups		anxiety management
		communication skills
		assertiveness
		relaxation

This section also details the various therapy approaches available to a PWS, specifically 'speak more fluently', stammer more fluently, 'stammer more proudly' and psychological approaches.

Approaches			
Speak more fluently	Stammer more easily	'Stammer more proudly'	Psychological approaches

44. THERAPY APPROACHES

It is important to differentiate between the various therapy approaches which are currently in use with adults who stammer.

i.   First, there are techniques designed to increase a person's level of fluency; this is the fluency modification or 'speak more fluently' approach. Fluency shaping focuses on the surface features of stammering: breathing, laryngeal and articulatory issues. Included here are strategies such as rate control, in which the person changes all of his speech pattern all of the time. There are other techniques such as easy onset which are applied to certain aspects of his speech, in this case using a modified start to an utterance, but, again, the recommendation is that this be used continuously. (See **Section F.**)

ii. Next, there are techniques which modify the nature of the dysfluency. This is the stammering modification or 'stammer more easily' approach. Here techniques such as block modification change the pattern of stammering to a less tense, struggle-free mode of speaking. The aim is not to remove the stammering but to create a form of dysfluency that is open and easy. In this approach, the PWS is required to evaluate and change his stammering in the moment it occurs. The remainder of his speech is not modified; only the periods of dysfluency are altered. (See **Section G.**)

iii. Psychological approaches. The primary goal of these approaches is described by Manning (2001) as changing:

"the way in which the client considers himself and his stuttering and how he interprets the events of stuttering."

(p. 276)

This can involve little direct speech modification but specific psychological interventions such as cognitive behavioural therapy (CBT) (Beck 1993), personal construct therapy (PCT) (Kelly 1955) and acceptance and commitment therapy (Harris 2009). (See **Section I.**)

iv. Social model. In recent times, there has emerged an approach based on the social model of disability. This has been called 'stammer more proudly'. In this approach, the individual is encouraged to claim his right to stammer and challenge the negative attitudes of society to stammering.

The following **Points 45–49** (i.e. effective therapy, principles of stammering therapy, prerequisites, openness and desensitisation) relate to therapy that can be used with any of the three approaches described previously. **Points 48–51** (i.e. openness, desensitisation, voluntary stammering and avoidance reduction) are relevant to stammer modification/stammer more easily and **Points 48, 50 and 51** (i.e. openness, voluntary stammering and avoidance reduction) for 'stammer more proudly'.

45. EFFECTIVE THERAPY

Before continuing to look at therapy options, it is important to consider what effective therapy should entail. There are a number of opinions on this. First, the World Health Organisation (WHO) advocates a multidimensional model of human

> I wish I knew that the treatment success should not be measured by the decrease or disappearance of dysfluencies, but rather by the degree of satisfaction reached by the patient and his overall quality of life.
> Selma Saad (Personal Communication 2021)

health, including concepts of 'impairment', 'activity limitation' and 'participation restrictions' This model has been used to evaluate the consequences of stammering (Yaruss & Quesal 2004). Using the WHO recommendations, any approaches to treating stammering should affect both the impairment and meaningfully change the limitations or restrictions of the problem, that is, the overt aspect of stammering and the covert elements, such as anxiety, shame and stigma.

"stuttering treatments should only be considered
successful if they reduce stuttering frequency (impairment level) and also reduce 'participation restrictions
or activity limitations'."

(Blomgren 2013, p. 15)

Second, those embracing the social model of disability and
the 'stammer more proudly' approach (see **Section H**) would
include a different set of outcomes; including:

"saying what you want when you want spontaneously,
sharing joy in connection and communication and
feeling confident as an equal partner in communication."

(Everard 2021)

In a recent conference presentation, Siskin stated that in the
future:

"Success in speech therapy will no longer be based in
looking neurotypical but on developing self-advocacy
and pride in one's identity, confidence and effectiveness in communication."

(2021)

Finally and perhaps most importantly, we should consider the
views of those who stammer. Plexico et al. (2005) carried out
a qualitative study to understand how stammering can be successfully managed from the perspective of a PWS. Six recur-
ring themes were identified as important for individuals who
stammered in the transition from unsuccessful to successful
management of stammering. These were:

- support from others, including counselling, self-help/
support groups, family and friends
- successful therapy, which provided behavioural and cognitive and emotional strategies to change both fluency
levels, and the feelings they (PWS) had about themselves
as speakers

- self-therapy and behavioural change, including risk taking and self-disclosure
- cognitive change, including risk taking, reduced fear of failure, taking responsibility for their speech, learning about themselves as a speaker and adopting a positive attitude
- utilisation of personal experiences, such as recognising positive attributes and strengths they had used in the past
- high levels of motivation/determination to succeed.

The process that led to successful management of stammering was summarised by the authors in this way:

> "Transitioning from a life dominated by the theme of stuttering to one in which stuttering was successfully managed required both cognitive and behavioral changes. Successful management of stuttering occurred gradually resulting in stuttering becoming a minor, rather than a dominant theme. Ongoing motivation and persistence resulted in finding help in many forms, particularly from mentors . . . who provided support and guidance. Although no particular treatment protocol or technique was associated with success, taking advantage of this help resulted in acceptance and taking responsibility for change. Accomplishments in many other areas were employed as counter themes to the perceived lack of ability to communicate successfully. Change is evident not only in the reduction of stuttering frequency, but in the ability to disclose the problem and take risks regarding communication outside of the treatment setting."
>
> (p. 14)

46. PRINCIPLES OF STAMMERING THERAPY

The general principles of speech and language therapy apply to working with stammering in the same way as other speech disorders: establishment of a clear management plan, with targets or goals broken down into small achievable steps and built-in rewards or validations when these have been achieved.

There are, however, a number of components which are particularly relevant to therapy with a PWS. These will be outlined here before moving on to discuss the more specific aspects of therapy.

- Tailor made. This text focuses on therapy that is designed for an individual adult or young person who stammers. Consequently, each management plan will be different, designed for the individual's particular needs and his learning style, and will evolve to accommodate any additional issues the person wishes to consider. (I believe those therapists wishing to follow a pre-determined programme for their clients will find themselves clinically constrained and with a percentage of clients dissatisfied and dropping out of therapy.)

- Hypothesis testing. In stammering therapy, the client and clinician jointly formulate a hypothesis on which the management plan is based. For example, after a lifetime of avoidance, Ruben decided to come for therapy. He had built his fluency on a complex array of strategies: word substitution, situation avoidance and being aggressive in order to be fluent. The hypothesis that he tested out in therapy was that he could risk being dysfluent, manage his stammer and the consequences of stammering and be more himself (which was someone who was sensitive and kind).

> It is quite easy to speak fluently when you [sic a PWS] visit your SLT. It is much more difficult to transfer it to normal life. As a therapist I had to face my worries, leave my comfort zone and face the world together with my clients.
> Jan Dezort (Personal Communication 2021)

- Experimentation. In the past, therapy comprised activities which took place in the clinic room. The result of this limited approach was that individuals struggled to move the progress they made into their everyday lives. These days, plans are made in clinic, and the work is carried out by the PWS within the context of his everyday life. Therapy is designed around a series of experiments in which the person tries out alternative possibilities. These may relate to thoughts, feelings or specific behaviours. Some preparatory work and try outs can be carried out initially in clinic, but then significant experimentation takes place by the person in the settings of his home, work and leisure activities and will usually involve his partner, family, friends, work colleagues and so on. The results and implications of these experiments are subsequently discussed in sessions with the therapist and further evaluations developed as a consequence. Using such an approach, a person does not fail; rather, he learns from his experimentation and refines his change process accordingly.

Andy began his experiment by practicing open stammering in clinic with his therapist. He tried out easy stammering first, that is, stammering without tension or struggle, and then progressed to letting the more disruptive repetitions and blocks occur. Once he felt comfortable and able to manage the anxiety associated with stammering, he moved the experiment to situations at home involving his partner and in one-to-one encounters with a good friend with whom he played football. Andy learned that he was more conscious of his dysfluencies than his SOs were. His friend told him that he didn't notice them much and he was more interested in the conversation topic (usually a discussion on the merits of Manchester United's latest match!).

- Choice. As in the previous example, the key notion is choice. The individual ultimately should choose the approach taken in therapy or whether he needs therapy at all. As persons who stammer, Richter and St Pierre (2014) attest:

"We need to be given the choice of whether or not to receive speech rehabilitation. Dysfluency-positive and dysfluency-negative perspectives should always be offered before choosing long-term speech therapy. We contend that at any age multiple perspectives on dysfluency are an absolute necessity for autonomous choice regarding one's therapeutic options."

(Point 4 www.didistutter.org, website home page)

Then, within the framework of the agreed-upon approach, the PWS will choose his mode of experimentation. He may feel some gentle pushing and encouragement from the therapist and involved SOs, and perhaps in a group therapy context he will experience peer pressure. Nevertheless, ultimately, he selects the methodology of the experiment: the specific issues to be worked on, the goals, the type of experiment, where it is to take place, for how long, the number of times, with whom and so on. In this way, he has control; the experiment is his, designed by him and for him and not thought out or imposed by the therapist.

47. PREREQUISITES

It may be that before getting started on some key therapy issues, a PWS needs to work on other areas to enable him to engage with therapy. Let us consider some areas to think about with an individual.

i.   Support mechanisms (or, as the title of this series is Navigational Points, perhaps we should call them buoyancy aids!). Does the PWS have sufficient support in place for him to lean on during difficult phases of change and to celebrate with when he has achieved specific goals? One way for the therapist to help him in this regard is to put in place mechanisms to support him as he progresses. These safety nets can include enlisting the help of SOs to encourage and support and provide a sounding board to discuss and reflect on his experimentation. Developing this system of support is a good long-term strategy which will be useful once therapy has come to an end. It ensures the individual knows that stammering and any associated issues can continue to be openly discussed with those who are important to him.

Another way of ensuring the person is supported is by encouraging him to become a member of a local self-help group or stammering organisation (e.g. British Stammering Association/Stamma). More will be said about this in **Section K.**

ii. Prerequisite skills. There may be skills and competencies that a PWS needs in order to work towards particular goals. For example, before embarking on avoidance reduction, Gareth needed to be able to manage his anxiety. In clinic, he learned a breathing technique which enabled him to do this.

In the following section, a number of areas will be described which could be precursors to work on specific targets.

• Preparing for change. Does a PWS need to gain confidence in his ability to change? Some adults embarking on therapy may be sceptical about what they can achieve, having tried and failed in the past. Others are wary of making change and need to be gradually introduced to it. Preparing for change and carrying out loose experiments (i.e. unimportant, small changes) are ways of managing such situations. Such an exercise can be described as follows: A client is first encouraged to talk about a positive change he has previously made: what the change was, when and how he decided to make the change, how he went about it and what factors he thinks were important in being able to make this positive difference.

Next the PWS is asked to make a change to some unimportant part of his everyday life. This may relate to an aspect of his appearance or a particular daily routine he has. For example, an individual can choose to wear a different item of clothing, adopt a different hairstyle or vary the route he takes to work, what he eats for lunch, what time he gets up or goes to bed, how he brushes his teeth. The possibilities are numerous, but it is important that the individual make the choice for himself.

The results of these experiments are discussed in detail in clinic. The therapist will be interested in how the person selected the area of change, his thoughts and feelings before during and after the experiment, how successful he was and any role another person played in helping him maintain the change.

Both these discussions and experimentation introduce the idea of a hierarchy of challenge and set the scene for change.

- Anxiety management. Does the PWS need to be able to control his levels of anxiety before being able to do anything else? While an individual who

> 🏛 I wish I had understood the role of anxiety in stuttering. It was important for me to understand the difference between trait anxiety and state anxiety.
> Monica Rocha (Personal Communication 2021)

stammers is not anxious or nervous in general (Alm 2014), many experience anxiety associated with speaking situations (i.e. state anxiety). Others have a more diffuse state of anxiety as a result of stammering (i.e. trait anxiety). It can be that both types of anxiety prevent a person from engaging in therapy experiments. He needs to be able to control his feelings of panic in order to then focus on trying out something different. In this situation, teaching a client some way of managing his anxiety first is an important safety net. This could be:

- A mindfulness approach which centres the person in the here and now and being aware and just observing in a non-judgmental way what is going on in real time. In this way, he can reduce stress and anxiety. (Mindfulness will be discussed in detail in **Psychological Approaches, Section I.**)
- Grounding exercises are also effective in controlling anxiety, as they bring the individual's focus away from his feelings of anxiety to the present moment. One example is the 5-4-3-2-1 exercise in which the person identifies numbers of items in progressively decreasing amounts. For example, 5 things he can see in his immediate surroundings, 4 sounds he can hear, 3 things he can feel, 2 smells he is aware of and 1 taste he is experiencing.
- Anxiety control training (Snaith 1981; Turnbull & Stewart 2017) or tension control training (TCT) (Williams www.llttf.com [accessed 4th Feb 2021]) is a technique developed by psychiatrist Philip Snaith. It incorporates relaxation and cognitive therapy to enable an individual to control visualised anxiety.

This has been proven to generalise to state and trait anxiety experienced by adults. Williams (2021) has a website called Living Life to the Full (www.llttf.com) which includes many resources, including free digital audio on anxiety control training/TCT, and these are useful to utilise and/or recommend to clients.

○   A simple breathing technique. The breathing square, or box breathing, is an example of something that can be easily taught and is effective for the client. As the name implies, the technique has the image of a square or a box at its centre. The person is instructed to sit comfortably and begins by gently inhaling through his nose for a count of four seconds. At the top of the inhalation, he pauses and gently holds the breath for four seconds. Next, he slowly exhales through his mouth for another four seconds and holds the empty lung state again for four seconds. He can be encouraged to visualise the track of the breath along the sides of a square: rising up one line of the square as he inhales; holding the breath across the top line, then down the other side of the square to exhale; and finally holding across the bottom line.

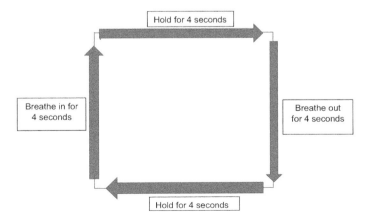

Figure 5.1 The Breathing Square

- ○ Relaxation. One common physical reaction to anxiety is muscle tension. Thus, exercises involving contrasting tense and relaxed muscle states can be useful for the PWS to identify which muscle groups are in tension when he experiences anxiety. He may then be able to work on inducing a more relaxed state, which will decrease his heart and breathing rate and thus reduce anxiety. This can be used in some settings but not all. Further discussion on relaxation can be found later in this section.
- Communication skills. Does a person need more effective communication skills before working on his stammering? Sometimes a PWS is so focused on his stammering behaviours (i.e. avoidance or duration of blocks) and his reactions (i.e. his fear of stammering, feelings of inadequacy) that he neglects the other aspects of communication which would make the exchange effective. For example, Penny started experimenting with speech modification work only to find she was unable to turn-take effectively and found it difficult to maintain a conversation. It is constructive to work on communication skills prior to key change experiments to ensure that these are in place and the outcomes of experiments are not determined by issues with communication.

    Key skills would include the following:
    - ○ Non-verbal communication (i.e. eye contact, facial expression, gesture, posture)
    - ○ Listening skills (i.e. active listening, use of affirmations, listening for content)
    - ○ Conversational skills (i.e. greetings, introducing topics, maintaining conversations, endings).

    A full description of appropriate communication skills training for adults who stammer, including several activities for use in one-to-one sessions and groups, can be found in Turnbull and Stewart (2017). Everard and Guldberg (2021) also discuss their focus on communication skills in a chapter on group therapy.

- Assertiveness training. Does a PWS need to be more assertive before working on his speech so that his voice is heard by others? Although there is some research which suggests assertiveness training can affect levels of fluency (Schloss et al. 1987), its use here is advocated as a safety net and not a fluency-enhancing technique.

  For example, Liu found it difficult to hold his own in conversations with his work colleagues. His contributions were ignored or passed over, and he was interrupted and generally felt undermined. In this situation, he felt the need for strategies which declared his right to speak, to have his turn and be listened to in the same way as other members of the group.

  Of relevance here are the following:
  - use of 'I' statements: 'I'm going to finish my comment'
  - rehearsal
  - repeated assertion, often called 'the broken record'
  - managing criticism, such as 'fogging' – acknowledging the criticism but holding onto your right to choose 'I agree that there are probably times when I don't look at you when you are talking. Sometimes it's because I'm thinking about what you are saying'
  - use of negative assertion, such as 'Yes, you're right. I don't always listen closely to what you have to say'
  - working on a compromise, for example, 'I understand that you want to talk to me now. However, I need to finish what I'm doing. So, give me five minutes and I'll sit down with you and talk then.'

Van Riper (1973) advocates the use of fixed role therapy (Kelly 1955) in teaching a PWS the role of an assertive speaker. He describes how a character sketch of an assertive person is written (Van Riper says it is written by the therapist, but I would suggest that the client write it and therefore take ownership of the sketch). The clinician will model the role in both the clinical setting and then later in real-life situations. Next the individual experiments with the role in the same situations, initially for a short period of time, moving to playing it out more continuously for several days.

A useful resource for clinicians wishing to develop assertiveness skills with a PWS is Nicholls (2009).

- Relaxation. Does the PWS's level of tension interfere with his ability to manage specific situations? As with assertiveness training, relaxation is not a treatment for stammering; rather, it is a safety net which helps a PWS to manage the difficult situations in which he fears and/ or experiences stammering. Manning (2001) wrote:

> "The goal [of relaxation] is not to promote fluency per se but to teach the client better ways of responding to stress-producing situations, whether giving a presentation to a large audience or having dental surgery."
>
> (p. 303)

There are three ways in which relaxation can be helpful:

- quick/in the moment relaxation techniques; such as scanning the body for sites of tension. Examples include:
  i.   sweeping the body with an imaginary soft brush
  ii. letting relaxation flow down the body from head to toes like a ripple
  iii. working through a number of postures the person knows help him to release tension in key parts of his body, such as head in the centre, shoulders down, arms loose, knees unlocked.

  Sometimes a client finds cognitive strategies a functional aid to his relaxation. Examples include the use of:
  i.   self-talk, e.g. 'I am calm and relaxed', 'I feel in control'
  ii. appropriate imagery, e.g. thinking of oneself as a ragdoll, a limp fleecy blanket or whatever works for the client.
- time-out techniques. These exercises involve an individual separating himself from everyday activities, usually in a quiet room, seated or lying down. They focus

on progressive muscle relaxation, that is, establishing a tension-free state in all muscle groups. Starting at the outer extremity, his toes or fingers, he works up through each major muscle group, flexing each one in turn for a count of ten seconds. This is followed by releasing the same group for a further count of ten seconds. He then moves onto the next group and repeats the flexion and release until all muscles have been engaged in this way.

- deep relaxation. This is a state of body and mind relaxation. It is achieved by carrying out the previous progressive relaxation technique (or some other method) while incorporating slow regular diaphragmatic breathing. Once a complete state of relaxation has been achieved, then the person quiets his mind and allows his focus to be on his breath alone. There are a number of audio or digital downloads available for clients to use at home for this purpose.

Common interventions (for use before a number of therapy approaches)			
Openness	Desensitisation	Voluntary stammering	Avoidance reduction

48. OPENNESS

An important issue to work on early in therapy is the PWS's ability to be open about his stammering. This is of benefit to the therapeutic dialogue but also helps in the development of more positive psychological responses to dysfluency.

> Stuttering is still a taboo here. Unfortunately, PWS adopt this view and they are isolated, lonely and that has a big influence on the way they see themselves.
> Jan Dezort (Personal Communication 2021)

Work on desensitisation, voluntary stammering and avoidance reduction should be carried out after focusing on openness.

Openness begins with experiments on making eye contact with people with whom the PWS is talking. In this way, he comes to see, literally, how people are reacting to his communication and challenges his pre-emptions about how others react to stammering. A client can start with people he feels comfortable with (i.e. family and friends) and then move to more challenging authority figures and those he regards as 'difficult listeners'.

Second, an individual should explore his own stammering behaviours and psychological responses through identification checklists, self-reporting, journal or diary keeping and so on. This may have been carried out as part of an assessment process, in which case it does not need to be repeated here.

Following on from this work, an individual is encouraged to explore stammering as a topic of conversation. Sheehan et al. (2005) talk about this in the context of a PWS accepting his role as a stammerer:

> "begin accepting your role as a stutterer by discussing stuttering with friends and acquaintances with whom you will be more tempted to show your stuttering."
>
> (p. 13)

Starting with those people he is comfortable with, a person can initiate a conversation in a number of ways:

- do you notice my stammering much?
- why do you think it happens?
- apart from me, do you know anyone else who stammers?

An individual will work up through a hierarchy of people from easy to most difficult. Then he can be challenged to carry out a short survey on stammering with members of the general public. This is a great exercise for groups but can be daunting for a PWS at the start of therapy to carry out on his own. One way of doing the survey as an individual is to enlist the support of another client currently undergoing therapy or member of a local self-help group to carry out the survey alongside him. This can be the start of a supportive relationship with another PWS and/or local self-help group.

Examples of questions which can be used are:

- personal knowledge of stammering: Do you have any friends or relatives who stammer? Have you ever met anyone who stammers? Do you know what stammering is?
- ideas about causation: What do you think causes stammering? Is stammering medical, psychological or some other sort of problem? What sort of people stammer?
- ideas about treatment: What do you think can be done about stammering? What treatment is available? Have you heard of speech and language therapy for individuals who stammer?
- feelings about stammering: What do you do when speaking to someone who stammers? What do you think is the most helpful way of reacting?
- social model: Do you think PWS experience negativity in society? Is a PWS disadvantaged because of the way he speaks?

(Turnbull & Stewart 2017, p. 112)

Linklater (2021) also advocates the use of this type of survey. His clients use a questionnaire which has some similar and slightly different questions.

Being open about stammering is a strategy which should be maintained beyond therapy. A PWS will feel more relaxed and in control if he introduces himself and his stammer to others almost in the same breath. If he continues to mention aspects of stammering period-ically with friends and family,

> There has been a long trad-ition in the Czech Republic that parents do not speak with children about their problems in speech. Stuttering is still a taboo here. Unfortunately, PWS adopt this view and they are isolated, lonely and that has a big influence on the way they see themselves. When we include this topic in public debate, including family, school and the whole society then it will help all PWS use their potential to maximum level.
> Jan Dezort (Personal Com-munication 2021)

it will lose its stigma and becomes less of a taboo topic which no one ever mentions or is hidden from sight. He may reach a point where he is able to accept his role as expert and become an advocate for stammering and the stammering community. (More about this role can be found in **Section H**.)

49. DESENSITISATION

Van Riper (1973) describes the principal objective of desensitisation:

> "to reduce the intensity of the attendant emotion enough so that the behavior becomes manageable."
>
> (p. 274)

This process is based on the belief that stammering is, in some part, a result of a person's reaction to it, that is, what you do to stop stammering. A young non-fluent child can be observed to move from easy repetitions to breath holding and blocks due to an increase in his awareness and sensitivity to dysfluency. We also notice the development of the 'under the surface' or covert attributes of stammering, such as shame, guilt, anger and frustration, as a result of a person's sensitive responses to his stammering.

The importance of desensitisation in any therapeutic approach for a PWS is crucial.

> "Desensitisation is seen as an essential and major part of most therapeutic interventions and is crucial to the maintenance of change."
>
> (Turnbull & Stewart 2017, p. 107)

It is however, a difficult and challenging undertaking for many individuals who stammer and needs to be carried out with care, understanding and the necessary time. It is vital that the process be explained fully to a client, including the rationale behind it, and to alert him to the likelihood that his overt or observable stammering behaviours may increase, at least for a time. A clinician should be courageous enough to stammer like her client in clinic and outside to demonstrate her own tolerance of dysfluency. Desensitisation necessitates open stammering; stripping away the strategies which the individual has used to hide it in the past. Consequently, stammering will be in full view, and increasing a person's tolerance of its appearance is one of the stages in this therapy.

Van Riper (1973, p. 274) described three areas to work on:

- confrontation of the dys-fluency: stammering openly, eliminating hiding strategies
- increasing a person's toler-ance for 'core stammering behaviours': being able to observe stammering in self and others without experien-cing negative reactions
- resisting communicative stress and listener penalty: being able to speak at one's own rate, manage interruptions, silences, requests for repetitions and other negative listener reactions.

> I wish I has more courage to accompany my patients in the desensitization phase when I began working with clients who stammered.
>
> I believe the desensitization phase is not very easy to be dealt with, and the SLP should be ready to approach it carefully with the patient, at the right time. I remember that 15 years ago I wasn't comfortable at all when using/modeling voluntary stuttering for example, while now I do it with much more confidence.
>
> Selma Saad (Personal Communication 2021)

Ideas for confrontation of stammering include:

- talking about personal experiences of stammering behaviours to SOs
- talking about the emotions associated with stammering to SOs
- talking about any stammering 'nightmare' scenario he might imagine to the therapist and SOs
- watching examples of types of stammering and carrying out analytical exercises such as the number of repetitions/prolongations heard in the examples
- taking a video of self while talking and watching it back with the support of a therapist and then with SOs.

Ideas for increasing tolerance of core stammering behaviours include:

- acknowledging stammering and/or avoidance in the moment, that is, noticing the stammer and commenting on it to a communication partner, such as, 'I stammered then. I always find that word difficult to say', or, 'I would normally avoid saying this word because I stammer on it, but I'm going to give it a go today'
- freezing stammers, that is, holding onto the moments of stammering; duplicating repetitions, extending prolongations
- collecting stammers, that is, monitoring the occurrence of particular types of stammering and having a daily target of dysfluencies to attain
- taking video of self while stammering in different situations and watching it back with the therapist and then with SOs.

Ideas for resisting communication stress and listener penalty include exercises for:

- tolerance of silence
- tolerance of time pressure
- holding eye contact
- using pausing
- speaking to difficult listeners in a role play with others; roles played can include distracted listeners, those who interrupt or ask for repetitions, individuals with poor eye contact or who mimic stammering
- speaking circles (Glickstein 1999). This is a group activity in which the clinician takes an equal part. The group sits in a semi-circle, and each person takes his turn to stand in front of the group. For 30 seconds, he makes eye contact with the group members. At the end of this period, the person who is timing will indicate the time has elapsed and the person at the front can now choose to speak for the remaining time (e.g. one minute) or continue just to keep eye contact. After this second time period, he is give

a round of applause and some brief positive feedback about his communication/delivery (not the content of any speech he may have given). The speaker does not comment on the feedback other than acknowledging it and thanking the listener(s). Once everyone has had a turn, there is a second round in which the optional speaking section is extended (i.e. to two or three minutes) depending on the time available and size of the group.

Details of other exercises can be found in Turnbull and Stewart (2017), Everard and Guldberg (2021) and Linklater (2021).

50. VOLUNTARY STAMMERING

When introduced to a PWS, voluntary stammering is often greeted with bewilderment and confusion. Having presented for therapy to alleviate stammering behaviours, the clinician is now suggesting doing more of them. This paradoxical therapy is nevertheless a powerful strategy, especially, according to Levy (1987), for more interiorised or covert stammerers. It has many benefits for the PWS, which are:

> I wished I had known that it would be best to persuade a person to try stuttering deliberately because it's very useful (especially) if someone was really afraid to do so.
>
> I realize now that people who are not open to stuttering on purpose are often the people that need this the most. They need to get to know the types of stutters, to reduce their fear for it and in some way take control of their stuttering.
>
> Jo Van der Sypt (Personal Communication 2021)

- desensitisation
- realisation that he can choose to stammer overtly in a different way
- learning ways of stammering in a controlled manner
- feeling in control while stammering openly
- the creation of a degree of objectivity; being able to separate the self from the moment of stammering
- being able to focus on other aspects of communication while stammering, e.g. eye contact, listener reactions

- reducing the negative emotions associated with open stammering, e.g. anxiety, stress, guilt
- avoidance reduction, especially around sounds and words
- acceptance of the role of stammerer
- providing a bridge to modification of his stammering behaviours.

Alongside their clients, clinicians are often confused about what voluntary stammering entails. It can be mistaken for variation of the PWS's stammering, which is changing his particular method of overt stammering, a strategy that may come later. (See **Section G**.) So what exactly is voluntary stammering?

Sheehan and Voas (1957) list a number of criteria which characterise good voluntary stammering:

- good eye contact
- prolongation or slide on the first sound of the word
- gentle repetition or bounce on the first sound of the word*
- used on non-feared words
- used in an unhurried manner
- varied in length from word to word
- used with smooth release
- used with forward movement.

*Note: both Sheehan and Voas (1957) and Linklater (2021) advocate the use of the prolongation alone rather than both the bounce and the stretch. They believe the bounce prevents the forward movement of speech, which is an important criterion in the use of voluntary stammering.

Teaching voluntary stammering is carried out after a full explanation of the rationale and extensive discussions have taken place. The clinician should provide the PWS with relevant reading material to take away and discuss with family members and others.

It is also useful to ask an older (in therapy terms) client who has embraced voluntary stammering to come to a session and talk about his experiences with the technique, its advantages and disadvantages and any advice he might give.

The first step is for the therapist to demonstrate voluntary stammering, prolongations and repetitions in a one-to-one session with the individual. She can do this in reading, monologue, question-and-answer activities and finally in free conversation. As she

> My first experience when I stuttered voluntarily was that it enabled me to understand the feelings of the PWS. It also changed the position of a therapist-client into a partner-client which completely changed the dynamics of my work.
> Jan Dezort (Personal Communication 2021)

proceeds, she will comment on and draw the PWS's attention to a number of factors:

- her eye contact
- which type of voluntary stammer she has used: prolongation/slide or repetition/bounce
- why she made the choice of one type or the other
  (Here there needs to be a conversation about the types of speech sounds most appropriate for certain types of voluntary stammers, e.g. repetitions for plosives, nasals, fricatives and affricates, prolongations for fricatives, continuants, nasals, vowels.)
- the numbers of repetitions and length of the prolongations
- the pace and timing
- her light articulatory contact
- the choice of words, and so on.

This demonstration will then move outside the clinic, and the clinician will show the PWS how voluntary stammering can be used in everyday situations. For example, ordering in a café or restaurant or asking a person for the time or the way to a venue. The PWS can be directed to observe for listener reactions. This monitoring and any queries he has regarding the therapist's use of voluntary stammering can be discussed back in the clinic room.

Practice then moves to the client. He can rehearse his use with the therapist in reading, monologue, question-and-answer exercises and conversation in the same way as the therapist but for a longer period of time. The work here will refine his use of the technique and enable him to use both prolongation and bounce on appropriate sounds in non-feared words, at a slow pace, and with good eye contact. Next, he will devise a hierarchy of situations from easy to hardest in which to move his experimentation outside into his everyday life.

Some clinicians recommend a progression from prolongations and bounce to the use of voluntary stammering which imitates their own stammering. Byrd et al. (2016) studied the effects of voluntary stammering on affective, behavioural and cognitive components of stammering. They found that following the client's initial reticence to use voluntary stammering, greater benefits were achieved when the voluntary stammering more closely matched the person's actual stammering and when it was used outside a clinical setting.

It is important to talk to the individual about the feelings accompanying his use of voluntary stammering at various points in the process. The clinician can then monitor any increase in negative feelings, such as anxiety, and remind him of his 'safety nets' as required.

51. AVOIDANCE REDUCTION

> "For many who stutter, avoidance behaviors can be the most handicapping aspect of the disorder. Avoidance behaviors may lead to reduced social and occupational participation. Over time, avoidance behaviors may also lead to negative affective functioning such as feelings of loss of control, decreased mood, and increased anxiety."
>
> (Blumgart et al. 2010)

Avoidance is a frequent strategy used by individuals who stammer. At its heart is a fear and an anticipation of stammering. Why does stammering create so much anxiety that avoidance seems the only option? Talking to a PWS, he described the core of the fear as a dread of being out of control:

> "it's about feeling out of control in social situations. Like a dream where you are on a bus and you suddenly

realise you have forgotten to put on your trousers. It's that feeling of being out of control in terms of your own self presentation. All of us in any encounter seek to present ourselves in a particular light and then stammering comes along which completely disrupts that. While ever you are not accepting of yourself as a stammerer, then you are stuck with turning up at work naked!"

(MB)

This fear results in avoidance behaviours described by Sheehan (1975) and others at many different levels:

- sound (Logan & Sheasby 2007), e.g. omission of a feared sound in a word, using 'ums' and 'ers', swallowing, throat clearing
- word, e.g. substitution of a word for another which may be related or unrelated in meaning. This can also result in circumlocutions and word reordering
- speech, e.g. choosing to remain quiet rather than stammering openly in front of others
- situation, e.g. choosing not to engage in a particular speaking situation or more generally any situations which require talking in front of others
- feeling, e.g. not expressing particular feelings for example anger or gratitude, as this can result in 'letting one's guard down' and allowing stammering to happen
- relationship, e.g. refraining from issues relating to relationships, for example introducing oneself, initiating conversations with strangers, building and developing dialogue (e.g. asking and answering questions), activities which maintain relationships (e.g. follow-up telephone calls), affirming and supporting others
- self-role, e.g. not accepting oneself as a person who stammers (e.g. viewing one's actions and behaviours in terms of stammering) (Sheehan 1975). It is as if the person is seeing his life through a stammering lens, for example, 'I could never be a teacher because of my speech'

- intention to behave (Stewart 2012). This level goes beyond Sheehan's original idea, as individuals are choosing not to engage in a process and appear passive and unwilling to involve themselves in social behaviours. A client presenting with extreme forms of avoidance at different levels (i.e. word, speech, situation, feelings etc.) can show a lack of intention to act. He chooses not to act and not to speak if he anticipates stammering, does not place himself in any situation where he feels his fluency will be compromised, only relates to those who already know about his stammering and collude with his avoidances and may appear depressed or to have given up.

These levels are not organised in a hierarchy. Single levels, such as word avoidance, can occur in isolation, but it is usual to see multiple levels of avoidance being used simultaneously. For example, a PWS who switches words may also have difficulty asking for specific items in shops or particular destinations at ticket offices for buses or trains. Consequently, he has both situational and word avoidance.

There are some individuals who have built their life around complex avoidance behaviours and as a result may appear quite fluent to an untrained observer. They may be referred to as covert (Starkweather 1987) or interiorised stammerers. (Douglass & Quarrington 1952).

Sometimes a client or SO might ask the perfectly valid question: What is wrong with avoiding something if it is too difficult and you can stop stammering by circumventing it? The answer is that there is nothing wrong with minor/occasional avoidance. It becomes a problem, however, when the person is compromising the way he wishes to behave and wishes to be or become because of choosing avoidance. For example, not saying what he wants to say when he wants to say it, not going into all situations and taking opportunities that life presents, not having the relationships and friendships he desires and not expressing his emotions or being fundamentally who he really is.

Each PWS coming to therapy will feel differently about the diverse levels of avoidance. So, it is imperative that the therapist ask him where it is best to start work to reduce these behaviours. Is it easier to reduce word substitution than tackle specific speaking situations, or will he find expressing one particular emotion, such as gratitude, the best place to start?

Once the PWS selects the level of avoidance to be worked on, then he should create his own hierarchy of experiments, in small, manageable steps, ranging from most feared at the top to least feared at the bottom, which will be the basis of his therapy. He then rates each item according to how fearful or distressing it would be to carry out the experiment.

Example of Eric's Word Avoidance Hierarchy

Word Avoidance Hierarchy		
Items in order (most feared to least feared)	Anticipated anxiety rating	Actual anxiety rating (scored immediately after the experiment)
After an avoidance, telling the person I'm talking to that I have avoided saying a word because I was worried about stammering.		1. 2. 3. 4. 5.
After any avoidance, working the feared word back into the conversation immediately and saying it again later in the day in another situation.		1. 2. 3. 4. 5.
Deciding on 10 (working up to 20) feared words each day and working them into various conversations at home, work and when meeting friends after work.		1. 2. 3. 4. 5.

(Continued)

(*Continued*)

Word Avoidance Hierarchy		
Items in order (most feared to least feared)	Anticipated anxiety rating	Actual anxiety rating (scored immediately after the experiment)
Saying (all) feared words as they come up when reading bedtime stories at home.		1. 2. 3. 4. 5.
Saying one feared word per day with a friend.		1. 2. 3. 4. 5.
Saying one feared word per day with my partner in conversation.		1. 2. 3. 4. 5.
Practicing saying feared words in therapy session.		1. 2. 3. 4. 5.

The PWS then starts to engage with the first item on his list, the one with the least amount of anticipated threat. This may be a roleplay with a therapist or SO or perhaps the person imagining himself in a specific situation in detail. The item can be repeated any number of times until the anxiety has reached a minimal level (as rated by the client) before moving onto the next item on his list.

In summary, the keys to working on avoidance are experiments based on individual hierarchies, with the PWS taking small steps which are repeated numerous times until his anxiety is reduced to a manageable level.

REFERENCES

Alm, P.A. (2014). Stuttering in relation to anxiety, temperament, and personality: Review and analysis with focus on causality. *Journal of Fluency Disorders*, 40, 5–21.

Beck, A.T. (1993). *Cognitive Therapy & the Emotional Disorders*. New York: Penguin.

Blomgren, M. (2013). Behavioral treatments for children and adults who stutter: A review. *Psychology Research & Behavior Management*, 6, 9–19.

Blumgart, E., Tran, Y. & Craig, A. (2010). Social anxiety disorder in adults who stutter. *Depression & Anxiety*, 27, 7, 687–92.

Burgess, S. (2019). www.health.org.uk/improvement-projects/delivering-speech-and-language-therapy-through-telemedicine-to-adults-who-stammer [Accessed 2 August 2021].

Byrd, C.T., Gkalitsiou, Z., Donaher, J. & Stergiou, E. (2016, August 1). The client's perspective on voluntary stuttering. *American Journal of Speech-Language Pathology*, 25, 3, 290–305.

Douglass, E. & Quarrington, B. (1952). The differentiation of interiorized and exteriorized secondary stuttering. *Journal of Speech & Hearing Disorders*, 17, 377–385.

Everard, R. (2021). *Report on Stuttering Treatment within the Social Model of Disability; Resolving Contradictions and Double Messages*. A presentation by Vivian Siskin at the Oxford Dysfluency Conference January 2021, Signal.

Everard, R. & Guldberg, C. (2021). Working together: The power of the therapeutic group. In T. Stewart (ed.), *Stammering Resources for Adults and Teenagers: Integrating New Evidence into Clinical Practice*. London: Routledge, Taylor & Francis Group.

Glickstein, L. (1999). *Be Heard Now! Tap into Your Inner Speaker and Communicate with Ease.* New York: Broadway Books.

Harris, R. (2009). *ACT Made Simple.* Oakland, CA: New Harbinger Publications Inc.

Kelly, G.A. (1955). *The Psychology of Personal Constructs.* New York: Norton.

Levy, C. (1987). Interiorised stuttering: A group therapy approach. In C. Levy (ed.), *Stuttering Therapy: Practical Approaches.* London: Croom Helm.

Linklater, J. (2021). Principles of avoidance-reduction therapy. In T. Stewart (ed.), *Stammering Resources for Adults and Teenagers: Integrating New Evidence into Clinical Practice.* London: Routledge, Taylor & Francis Group.

Logan, J. & Sheasby, S. (2007). Using therapeutic writing to support a client's new story. *Signal,* 27, 2–3.

Manning, W.H. (2001). *Clinical Decision Making in Fluency Disorders.* Canada: Singular Thompson Learning.

Nicholls, S. (2009). *Let's Talk Assertiveness.* London: Routledge, Taylor & Francis Group.

Plexico, L., Manning, W.H. & DiLollo, A. (2005). A phenomenological understanding of successful stuttering management. *Journal of Fluency Disorders,* 30, 1–22.

Richter, Z. & St Pierre, J. (2014). Did I stutter? Project. www.didistutter.org [Accessed 2 August 2021].

Schloss, P.J., Freeman, C.A., Smith, M.A. & Espin, C.A. (1987). Influence of assertiveness training on the stuttering rates exhibited by three young adults. *Journal of Fluency Disorders,* 2, 5, 333–335.

Sheehan, J. (1975). Conflict theory and avoidance-reduction therapy. In J. Eisenson (ed.), *Stuttering: A Second Symposium.* New York: Harper Row.

Sheehan, J.G. & Voas, R.B. (1957). Stuttering as conflict: Comparison of therapy techniques involving approach and avoidance. *Journal of Speech & Hearing Disorders,* 22, 5, 714–723.

Sheehan, V.M., Shanks, P. & Mereu, S. (2005). *Easy Stuttering: Avoidance-Reduction Therapy.* Santa Monica, CA: Sheehan Stuttering Center.

Siskin, V. (2021, January). *Stuttering Treatment within Social Model of Disability; Resolving Contradictions and Double Messages*. Presentation at the Oxford Dysfluency Conference, Oxford.

Snaith, R.P. (1981). *Clinical Neurosis*. Oxford: Oxford University Press.

Starkweather, C.W. (1987). *Fluency & Stuttering*. Englewood Cliffs, NJ: Prentice-Hall Inc.

Stewart, T. (2012). Avoidance in adults who stammer: A review and clinical discussion. *Polish Forum Logopedyczne*, 20, 20–29.

Turnbull, J. & Stewart, T. (2017). *The Dysfluency Resource Book*, 2nd edition. London: Routledge, Taylor & Francis Group.

Van Riper, C. (1973). *The Treatment of Stuttering*. Englewood Cliffs, NJ: Prentice-Hall, Inc.

Williams, C. (2021, February). Tension control training [online]. www.llttf.com [Accessed 4 February 2021].

Yaruss, J.S. & Quesal, R.W. (2004). Stuttering and the international classification of functioning, disability, and health: An update. *Journal of Communication Disorders*, 37, 1, 35–52.

OTHER RESOURCES

Avoidance Reduction Therapy in a Group Setting. (Vivian Siskin). In this 2-hour DVD, Vivian Siskin 'walks clinicians through methods of group therapy while providing the nuts and bolts of Avoidance Reduction Therapy'. As well as a tutorial for SLTs, the DVD can serve as a self-primer for a PWS.

Fluency shaping vs stuttering modification by Uri Schneider. Available on YouTube: Schneider Speech.

Message to a Stutterer and No Words to Say. This DVD includes 'Message to a Stutterer' (34 minutes), a documentary tribute to eminent American psychologist Joseph Sheehan, who ran the stammering clinic at the University of California for 35 years. It comprises archive footage of research, experimentation, lectures and TV appearances outlining avoidance reduction therapy. In 'No Words to Say' (56 minutes), filmed at UCLA's stammering clinic, students share their personal experiences: their fears, failures and triumphs.

Fluency shaping vs stuttering modification by Uri Schneider. Available on YouTube: Schneider Speech.

Section F

THERAPY

Fluency modification or 'speak more fluently' approach

52. USING MULTIPLE STRATEGIES

Fluency modification has been described concisely by DeNil and Kroll (1995):

> "The basic premise of this approach is that stuttering is a physical behavior that can be modified by systematic exposure to a series of rules for fluent speech. The specific and observable behaviors of speech that are reconstructed include those related to speech rate, respiration, voice onset and articulation. Clients are provided with specific instructional sets for individual response units initially taught in isolation. These responses are then transferred gradually to more complex sequences and ultimately to conversational speech."

This technique was introduced in the 1960s by Goldiamond (1965), who demonstrated that a PWS could attain fluent speech using this speech pattern.

Following this early work, fluency modification has been taught using a multiple strategy approach. Several techniques have been combined in order for a PWS to adopt a different manner of speaking than his own dysfluent way. This speech, sometimes called smooth or slowed speech, combines:

- light articulatory contacts
- prolongation of sounds

DOI: 10.4324/9781003177890-7

- easy onset or gentle starts
- rate control
- regular, relaxed breathing. (Unlike **Section E, Point 47**, where a breathing technique is used to manage anxiety, here the issue is how it might be linked to stammering events and how modifications to a person's respiration can enhance his levels of fluency.)

Blomgren (2013) described the combination of techniques as speech restructuring:

> "Speech restructuring refers to speech therapy where a client is taught to use a new speech pattern. These approaches are also called 'fluency shaping' or 'prolonged speech' treatments. Slowed or prolonged speech is typically the primary component of any new speech pattern. The person who stutters is also taught to make speech motor movements with less articulatory pressure and to initiate vocal fold vibration in a gradual and controlled manner. The premise is that stuttering speakers habitually use speech production strategies that are outside their speech motor control abilities. The goal of speech restructuring is to promote a new speech production pattern that is conducive to fluent speech."
>
> (p. 14)

By using all of these techniques together, a PWS is able to eliminate his dysfluent speech but at the cost of a markedly different type of speech, which some listeners might say sounds unnatural.

> I wish I had known how much energy it takes to use techniques and how hard it is for PWS to use them and be able to concentrate.
> Jeanette Zammit (Personal Communication 2021)

Work is then needed to naturalise these patterns to a more normal-sounding speech while retaining the elements which maintain fluency. The other important consideration in the use of this approach is that it has to be used all the time; every time the PWS speaks, in every situation and with every person, he is expected to speak using these strategies. This is a very difficult task. However, it can be done, and I have known clients who embraced smooth speech and managed to make it sound natural. Nevertheless, it requires extreme focus and determination and is often too demanding for clients.

Brendan was referred by his GP when he was in his early 20s and job hunting. At that time, he wanted to eliminate his dysfluencies in order, as he saw it, to make himself more employable. He learnt to use a modified form of prolonged speech with additional work on diaphragmatic breathing and was able to speak fluently in clinic and other controlled conversations outside the clinic setting. He was seen periodically after that and reported using these techniques when he needed to but not all the time. Brendan returned to therapy some time later, when he was expecting his first child. On this occasion, he wanted to refresh his use of his fluency strategies, especially in reading. He was already anticipating stammering in front of his unborn child and wished to ensure he could read a bedtime story fluently. Although we did work in the way he initially requested, it became clear that his real reason for seeking therapy was to discuss with me the possibility that his child may have a stammer and how he might manage such a situation should it arise. I talked to him about what we knew about the heredity of stammering but also reminded him that this baby was being born to one of the best experts in stammering. The baby would be in the best place should its speech be dysfluent. (The story continued as the child did experience some dysfluencies from the age of four years, and Brendan and his wife came to sessions to work on creating the best environment for him.)

Although slowed speech is more associated with therapy of some decades ago, interestingly, the Camperdown Programme (O'Brian et al. 2010) currently in use in Australia, has many similarities with slowed speech. In this programme, a PWS is taken through four separate stages:

i.   an introduction to the prolonged speech technique (see **Point 56**)

  ii.   practice of the technique in clinic to achieve fluent and natural-sounding speech
  iii. generalisation of the technique to outside clinic speaking environments
  iv.   maintenance of fluent speech on an ongoing basis in everyday speaking situations.

O'Brian et al. (2010), reporting on the outcomes of the programme, stated that many adults were able to control their dysfluencies using prolonged speech; however, longer-term maintenance in everyday situations was proving more challenging.

It should also be noted that in the purest form, the 'speak more fluently' approach addresses only the surface or overt features of stammering using a behavioural modification method. Time is not given to the consideration of any psychological or emotional responses to stammering a PWS might have. The assumption is that fluency will provide the answer to the individual's concerns. As such, this approach may not prove enough for a PWS, and additional work on other issues may be needed. However, a person will need to reach that conclusion in his own time, perhaps after having experienced the fluency-shaping programme for himself.

Mo was a young man who referred himself for therapy, wanting a more fluent way of speaking. He felt that his stammer held him back in his role in the bank. In therapy, he worked on a number of fluency-enhancing strategies and was able to speak without stammering in clinic using these techniques. However, he struggled to maintain this way of talking outside clinic. One evening, at the end of a group session, we were walking out of the clinic together to the car park, and I commented to him that he wasn't using the techniques he had demonstrated only a few minutes previously. He said, 'Well, it just doesn't feel like me when I speak like that.' He went on to describe how the fluency he was able to achieve seemed to inhibit his natural communication and self-expression. Although he had thought fluency would give him the speech he wanted, in fact, what he wanted now was a more spontaneous communication style.

His objective had changed, having had the experience of using a controlled speech pattern.

53. TARGETING STRATEGIES

An alternative method is to look at which strategy or strategies are most effective for the client's particular stammer. One area which I recommended assessing in **Section D, Point 40** was the level of breakdown of the stammer. The PWS can experience a breakdown of his speech pattern at:

- articulatory/oral level
- phonatory/laryngeal level
- respiratory/diaphragmatic level.

The fluency-enhancing techniques can be matched to the level of breakdown, as summarised in the following table:

	Level of breakdown		
	Articulatory/ oral	Laryngeal	Respiratory/ diaphragmatic
Light contacts	☺		
Prolongation of sounds	☺	☺	
Easy onset	☺	☺	☺
Rate control	☺	☺	☺
Breathing		☺	☺

54. TEACHING FLUENCY MODIFICATION STRATEGIES

After each technique has been explained and demonstrated by the therapist, the person will experiment with it at a single sound level in clinic. The extension of the use of each technique is then carried out using a method called GILCU: gradual increase in length and complexity of utterance. It is important that this work not be confined to the therapy room but practised in everyday settings. The order of GILCU practice, with examples, is detailed in the following:

- simple monosyllabic words at CV and CVC level, examples are ink, hair, nose, jam, cheap, time
- more complex single words, including consonant clusters, that is, CCVC, CCCV, CCVCC, CCCVCCC, examples are clap, strain, brink, squirrel, strengths
- polysyllabic words, e.g. national, industrial, amalgamation, responsibility
- phrase level, e.g. 'fish and chips', 'the weather man'
- short sentences, e.g. 'Where are you?' 'A cup of coffee, please.'
- question-and-answer exchanges, e.g. 'Where do you live?' 'I live in Yorkshire. Where do you live?' 'I used to live in Yorkshire but now live outside Manchester.'
- longer sentences with adverbial, adjectival clauses, e.g. 'The football team wearing a black and white striped kit plays at St James' Park in Newcastle.'
- multiple sentences, e.g. 'On Saturday, I went to the supermarket and had lunch in a local café. When I got back home, as it was such a sunny day, I decided to go for a walk.'
- monologue and/or picture descriptions
- conversation that is spontaneous or centred around a selected topic.

55. LIGHT CONTACTS

This technique addresses the way in which a person articulates consonant sounds. Often a PWS uses a hard articulatory attack when producing sounds as part of his stammering pattern, for example, tensing his tongue against his alveolar ridge, pushing the contact with excessive force and using too much air pressure. The aim of this strategy is to counter the hard attack with a focus on articulating with minimum pressure and tension.

Teaching: When teaching such an activity, a clinician should first make sure that the PWS understands the mode of articulation of consonants. Time should be spent, with appropriate visual aids, explaining the various ways sounds are produced, particularly nasal versus oral sounds and the different places of articulation which are used in and around the mouth.

The therapist should introduce light contacts on single sounds in this order:

- approximants, continuants, liquids
- nasals
- fricatives and affricates
- plosives

She should demonstrate production at a single sound level, including contrasting hard and soft attack and having the PWS discriminate between the two. Once he is clear about the difference, the PWS can experiment as he feels able. It is important to give him feedback but more important to develop his own monitoring skills. Thus, I suggest always asking the individual how he thought his practice was before giving therapist feedback.

Once light contact is established on each sound, practice can proceed using the GILCU method described in **Point 54**.

Potential difficulties and some solutions: Clients rarely have difficulty with this technique, but where they do, it is usually as a result of:

- poor discrimination of hard and soft attack and/or
- lack of monitoring of their contacts.

These issues can be remedied with exercises on discrimination of hard and soft attack in the therapist's speech and others, such as SOs. This should be followed by contrasting productions in the PWS's own speech at a single sound level and in mono- and polysyllabic words. Monitoring can be improved by recording the individual speaking in clinic and in every day settings and then listening back. The recorded examples can be analysed,

especially instances of articulatory attack on the specific sounds
the PWS finds problematic.

56. PROLONGATION OF SOUNDS

Also regarded as a feature of stammering, sound prolongation,
paradoxically, may be used to enhance fluency. This is especially
the case when a PWS experiences difficulties in transitioning
from one sound to another.

Prolongation of sounds was the primary feature of a fluency modification technique in the 70s and early 80s called
prolonged speech. A client learning this technique was taught
to slightly prolong the vowels across his whole utterance. The
resulting speech, with its reduced melody and even stress
pattern, was not acceptable as natural fluency and rejected by
many clients. Consequently, the technique was modified to
include prolongations of both consonants and vowel sounds.
This sounded slightly better but, again, required additional
efforts after the initial learning phase to improve its accept-
ability as a speech pattern.

I include it here for completeness but also because it has a
place with some individuals whose stammer occurs:

- between word boundaries
- after a breath
- in the middle of words.

Teaching: The therapist should teach prolongation of sounds in
order from the easiest to prolong to the hardest. The recommended
order is:

- vowels
- approximants, continuants, liquids
- nasals
- fricatives and affricates
- plosives

Note: with regard to plosives, by their nature, it is difficult to
release a plosive in a prolonged or stretched way. Consequently,

it is necessary to explain the inherent features of a plosive and how it is produced. The therapist can then demonstrate how to shorten the stop phase and prolong the release phase and help the PWS to replicate this manner of production. (This way of articulating a plosive obviously affects the quality of the sound, but this is temporary and only really apparent at an early stage when the sound is being produced much slower than normal.)

Rather than teaching prolongation of sounds and vowels across all speech, clinically I have found it more appropriate for an individual to prolong the initial phoneme of a breath group (and consonant cluster), sliding into the sound. Following this initial prolongation, the rest of the utterance can be spoken in the usual way. It is useful to slow speech production down while in the early stages of learning this technique. Once it has been mastered, then normal speech rate can be reintroduced. By using this modified approach of only prolonging an initial sound, the person does not lose his normal intonation and melody of his voice, and the additional naturalising exercises should not be required.

Potential difficulties and solutions: On occasion, an individual may adopt a particular intonation pattern alongside the prolongation of the initial sound, for example, stressing the first syllable of the word in addition to the stretching of the first phoneme; '**The** team lost on Saturday.' '**My** favourite colour is blue.' The result can be a rather unusual speech pattern which will need further work. In order to avoid this occurring, a client should be encouraged to carry out some experimentation with different stress patterns at the sentence level. Examples of such an experiment are given in the following:

(The stressed word is indicated by the underline)

Example 1. Instructions: 'Use an easy start on the first word but emphasise the underlined words.'

- The best film you should watch tonight is one which has a good story and great acting.
- The best film you should watch tonight is one which has a good story and great acting.
- The best film you should watch tonight is one which has a good story and great acting.

Example 2. Instructions: 'Use an easy start on the first word but emphasise the underlined words.'

- There are <u>green</u> and <u>blue</u> curtains behind the sofa in the <u>old</u> house.
- There are green and blue <u>curtains</u> behind the <u>sofa</u> in the old house.
- There are green and blue curtains <u>behind</u> the sofa in the <u>old</u> house.
- There <u>are</u> green and blue curtains behind the sofa in the old <u>house</u>.

57. EASY ONSET

Gentle or easy onset has been a feature of many programmes in the past used with both children and adults who stammer (Gregory 1991; Runyan & Runyan 1993; Shine 1988; Shapiro 1999). In these instances, it appears as part of a multi-strategy approach which often includes breathing, relaxation, light articulatory contacts and rate control. I have used it in the same way but also as a stand-alone technique for clients who demonstrate a breakdown of fluency at the respiratory/diaphragmatic and/or laryngeal level. A clinician may observe the PWS has specific issues such as:

- significant difficulty with coordinating exhalation and onset of phonation
- blocks at the beginning of an utterance
- hard vocal attack.

(In some instances, there can be an additional breakdown at the articulatory level with the individual speaking with tense or hard articulatory contacts.)

Teaching: The technique is relatively simple and involves teaching a PWS to co-ordinate his exhaled air and the first sound of his utterance. Before starting, the PWS should be relaxed, especially in his chest, neck and mouth, and he must be able to use a diaphragmatic breathing pattern. (See **Point 59**.)

The instructions for the technique are as follows:

- Take a normal relaxed breath in. (Note: Do not hold the air at the top of the inhalation.)
- Gently exhale a small amount of air. (It is useful to demonstrate this as a flow of air, rather than blowing out air or emitting a puff of breath.)
- Once the flow of air is initiated, then begin to say the first sound of the utterance.
- Slightly extend the length of the articulatory contact for the sound, e.g. 's..hop', 'l..ight', 'a..pple'. (Note: this is not a repeated sound but a prolonged sound.)

This single-phoneme practice should be carried out in the same specific order as specified for prolonged sounds (see **Point 56**), and exercises will proceed using the GILCU plan (see **Point 54**). It is worth noting that in consonant clusters, it is only the initial consonant that is prolonged, for example, T – rudy, not Tr – udy.

Potential difficulties and solutions: There are a number of frequently occurring problems a PWS can experience when learning this technique. For example:

- In relation to breathing: breath holding at the top of the inhalation, blowing air out before beginning to say the sound (this may sound like the client is saying 'h'), letting out too much exhaled air.

  In this case, it is important to revise or return to the breathing explanation and practice.
- In relation to coordination: taking too long to inhale, exhaling a small amount of air but then stopping before saying the first sound.

  Here a PWS will benefit from reviewing work on the phase of inhalation and the start of phonation with soft attack. The shortening of the inhalation time should be done gradually.
- In relation to tension: clavicular and/or diaphragmatic tension, hard attack on the initial phoneme, vocal cord

closure (laryngeal tension), rising inflection with onset of phonation, forceful exhalation/too much air pressure.

When tension is the issue, work on self-monitoring and discriminating the feelings of relaxation and tension are useful. These can be carried out in relation to the specific area of tension for the PWS, such as respiration, laryngeal function and/or articulation.

- Other areas: lack of prolongation of the first sound, prolongation of whole word rather than the first sound of the word.

Again, exercises contrasting the target production with other less helpful productions, including what the individual is using, are most relevant here.

58. RATE CONTROL

In discussing rate control with a PWS, I have often had a client carry out this exercise or discussed this analogy: If a person was to walk from point A to point B at a normal pace, then this could be timed to establish his walking rate. If he was then asked to walk the same distance but to use more time/a slower walking pace, he could achieve this in a number of ways:

- pausing deliberately after each step
- pausing after a group of steps
- slowing the time taken for each step: a sliding step or walking with the feet keeping contact with the ground.

Translating this into speech rate terms, rate can be slowed by:

- pausing after each word
- pausing to take a breath/at breath group markers
- slowing the rate of articulation of each sound by prolonging vowels and stretching the duration of each articulatory contact.

In the past, rate control was taught primarily using the latter method. Syllables were spoken to a strict timed duration, and this was increased incrementally. Blomgren (2013) describes the method in this way:

> "Decreasing speech rate is best achieved by stretching the duration of syllables, not necessarily by inserting longer pauses between utterances. Initially, speech is produced at a very slow rate. In the UUISC [University of Utah Intensive Stuttering Clinic] each syllable is prolonged for two seconds. After fluent speech has been established at 2-second stretch, syllable durations are systematically shortened to 1 second, 0.5 seconds, and finally to 'controlled normal rate.' Controlled normal rate is the rate that a person who stutters can speak with little or no stuttering. The final rate varies for each client."
>
> (p. 16)

Although many clients were able to maintain this in clinic and certain situations in which they could be very controlled, its transfer to more demanding and stressful situations was difficult. In addition, the resulting speech lacked variation and consequently spontaneity.

Teaching: A much more responsive way of teaching rate control is a method which is flexible to the PWS's:

- mood
- confidence
- natural speech pattern
- level of anxiety in relation to the words he wishes to use and/or the given situation
- perception of the person/people to whom he is speaking.

Thus, the rate used needs to be flexible and variable to suit the ebb and flow of these factors. I recommend teaching rate as a set of gears; gears are used on a car to vary the speed according to setting off, the need to slow due to road conditions, hazards, lack of driver confidence (i.e. not being able to see or predict what is ahead) and coming to a halt. In the same way, a speaker's speed of speech should be adjusted according to how he is feeling, his level of confidence, how he anticipates words, his need for breath and so on. A clinician needs to work on speed variation with the person using:

- pausing
- taking time to inhale air
- prolongation of words and/or sounds.

These are then used to establish with the PWS:

- a rate he can use when he is opening a conversation, saying his name, for example (i.e. first gear). This will be a slow and controlled rate, featuring some prolongated initial sounds on feared words.
- a rate he can use when he has passed the initial introductory phase. This will be a little faster than the early rate but include pauses for breath and prolongations when he needs them (i.e. second gear). It is a sort of feeling-the-way speed of talking.
- a rate he can use in open talking. In conversations where he has no fear of interruptions or difficult words, where he can concentrate on the content of his utterance and his listener(s) and good communication in general (i.e. fourth gear).

Unlike the rate control of the past, there will not be a set timed number of words or syllables for each of these rates. Rather, the therapist will help the person determine his individual optimal speed for these three gears and help him experiment with their use in different contexts.

Potential difficulties and solutions: Sometimes a PWS has difficulty controlling his speech rate because of a more general issue of living life at a very fast pace. In these instances, it will be necessary for him to experiment with varying the pace of non-speech behaviours. For example, adopting an eating style where he chews each mouthful slowly and carefully, walking slowly to a specific destination, brushing his hair or shaving more slowly.

Other adults may struggle due to difficulties tolerating silence, experiencing feelings of urgency or concern over losing speaking turns. In these occurrences, work on anxiety management, and diaphragmatic breathing can shift focus and calm worries.

59. BREATHING

If the PWS is observed and reports stammering at the respiratory/diaphragmatic level, then work on breathing should be carried out. Other than at the specific request of the client, there would be no other reason to work on breathing as a fluency strategy.

There are independent, non-SLT programmes for adults who stammer which are based on teaching a specific breathing technique. The aim of these programmes is for all participants to learn to breathe in a different way as a means of becoming fluent. Each person's fluency is assessed prior to beginning the course, but his breathing is not. (This issue relates back to the clinical premise of assessing the areas that therapy intends to change. (See **Section D, Point 41**, 'Outcome-Based Assessments'.) I can see how such courses are relevant for adults whose stammering is related to their breathing, but in the absence of evidence of, for example, incorrect diaphragmatic breathing, or clavicular breathing, I fail to see its relevance.

When assessing the respiratory level of breakdown in stammering, there are a number of important areas to consider:

- tension. Does his general posture lend itself to constricted or limited lung expansion, for example, in positions where the shoulders are hunched or the ribcage is hyperextended? Is the person showing significant tension in his shoulders and chest? Is his diaphragm held rigidly? It may be that work on reducing levels of tension will be enough to improve the individual's breathing pattern.
- breathing pattern. Assessment/observation must also include monitoring the individual's manner of respiration,

both at rest and during speech. In particular, a clinician should look at:

- o the depth of the PWS's breathing: is he demonstrating shallow and/or clavicular breathing, with shoulders lifted during inhalation, limited movement of the rib-cage and consequently reduced air entering the lower and larger parts of his lungs?

- o reverse breathing: if this is a factor, the individual's diaphragm will be moving outwards during exhalation and moving in during inhalation. (Note: the normal pattern is the reverse of this; the diaphragm moves out during inhalation to accommodate the expansion of the lungs and then moves inwards, pushing the lungs up and in to squeeze out the exhaled air.)

- o the function of the intercostal muscles. These muscles control the amount of air and rate at which it is inhaled and exhaled. If a PWS is asked to exhale while saying a continuous sound like /s/ or /l/, then the sound will be variable in volume or intensity if the intercostal muscles are weak or ineffective. Similarly, if he is instructed to inhale slowly, the intercostal muscles will help him control the pace of his in-breath.

- rate of breathing, that is, the time taken for each breath. This is different for speaking as opposed to respiration while the body is at rest. In breathing for speech, the inhalation time is shorter, and the exhalation time fits the length of the utterance or phrase. For a PWS, the inspiration time can be too short and not give him time to take in enough air. With regard to the exhaled air, in normal speaking, there is an interesting equivalency between the speaker's unit of meaning and the out-breath, and this 'matching of air to meaning' seems to happen automatically. A PWS can lack this correspondence in the unit of meaning and the exhaled air, to the extent that he will run out of air when trying to fit in the words he needs to.

- frequency, that is, the number of times a person breathes in and out. This is important, as a high frequency of respiration or over-breathing can result in hyperventilation. With regard to speaking, hyperventilation can reflect a PWS's level of anxiety in a given situation. A low frequency of inspiration will, again, result in the person running out of air while trying to speak.

- timing. When talking, a person will coordinate the beginning of his out-breath with the onset of his speech. In stammering, specifically blocking, there has been research on an apparent lack of co-ordination of the onset of voice and the exhalation, such that the larynx locks and the voicing fails to start, resulting in a freezing of the vocal tract (Weiner 1984; Williams & Brutten 1994). Thus, it is essential to assess the PWS's coordination of respiration and phonation.

- pressure. A therapist should assess whether her client is breathing too deeply. As Poburka (2002) describes, this can cause some problems in controlling the pressure under the larynx and result in speech with integral aspects of tension:

"Speakers who breathe too deeply before speaking create an excessive amount of relaxation pressure inside the chest. Relaxation pressure is the force that causes air to be released from the lungs on exhalation. When relaxation pressure is greater than the pressure requirements for voice and speech, the individual must somehow deal with the excess pressure. Some people manage the pressure by using the larynx as a flow regulator or valve trying to hold back the excessive pressure (Morrison & Rammage 1993). As a result, their speech is characterized by hard glottal attacks, excessive loudness, and a pressed quality. For individuals who stutter, this sort of breathing strategy could encourage laryngeal tension making it difficult to use a relaxed voice onset."

(www.mnsu.edu/comdis/isad5/papers/
poburka.html)

Teaching: There are three key components when teaching breathing to a client who stammers:

- explain the process of respiration fully and with visual aids when possible. McLaughlin (2021, p. 54) describes a useful explanation of voice production which includes what she calls the 'power system' (respiratory system) with a simple line drawing of head, neck and lungs.

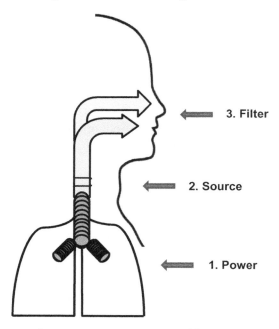

Figure 6.1 The Power System (McLaughlin 2021)

- work on capacity, that is, improving the amount of air which is taken in and moves out of the lungs. This can be done primarily by teaching diaphragmatic breathing, with appropriate:

- ○ relaxation
- ○ rate
- ○ frequency
- ○ pressure.

When using exercises to develop these aspects, the PWS ought to enhance his practice with visual and kinaesthetic feedback, such as watching himself in a mirror, looking for unnecessary tension and/or accessory movements of the shoulders and placing his hands on his ribs to monitor rib-cage movement and/or abdomen to monitor diaphragmatic function.

- • work on control, such as by decreasing tension (especially in the shoulders and diaphragm) and improving the function of the diaphragm and the intercostal muscles. Work should include specific exercises on shortening inhalation time, lengthening exhalation time and coordinating exhalation and phonation.

This can be done by speaking sentences of increasing length on one breath. For example:

He took her out for a meal.

He took her out for a meal last night.

He took her out for a meal last night to a local Italian restaurant.

He took her out for a meal last night to a local Italian restaurant they had not been to before.

He took her out last night to a local Italian restaurant they had not been to before even though he was feeling tired.

He took her out last night to a local Italian restaurant they had not been to before even though he was feeling tired having been to the gym earlier in the day.

Several useful breathing exercises can be found in Turnbull and Stewart (2017), Chapter 11.

Potential difficulties and solutions: These are summarised in the following table.

	Possible solutions					
	Tension reduction (maybe related to anxiety)	Diaphragmatic breathing	Breathing frequency	Diaphragm function	Intercostal function	Timing of exhalation and phonation or articulation
Tense posture	☺					
Shallow or clavicular breathing	☺	☺		☺	☺	
Poor intercostal movement	☺	☺			☺	
Diaphragm not moving/rigid	☺	☺		☺		
Rapid exhalation	☺		☺			
Air forced out	☺	☺			☺	☺
Running out of air	☺	☺	☺	☺	☺	
Over-breathing	☺				☺	
Variable volume of air on exhalation/inconsistent exhalation					☺	
Inspiration takes too long					☺	☺
Not inhaling often enough			☺		☺	☺
Reverse breathing		☺		☺		
Inhaling too much air					☺	☺

REFERENCES

Blomgren, M. (2013). Behavioral treatments for children and adults who stutter: A review. *Psychological Research & Behavioral Management*, 6, 9–19.

DeNil, L. & Kroll, R.M. (1995). The relationship between locus of control and long-term stuttering treatment outcome in adult stutterers. *Journal of Fluency Disorders*, 20, 345–364.

Goldiamond, I. (1965). Stuttering and fluency as manipulatable operant response classes. In I. Krasner & I. Ullmann (eds.), *Research in Behavior Modification*. New York: Holt, Rinehart and Winston.

Gregory, H.H. (1991). Therapy for elementary school-age children. *Seminars in Speech & Language*, 12, 323–335.

McLaughlin, A. (2021). Stammering & voice. In T. Stewart (ed.), *Stammering Resources for Adults and Children: Integrating Evidence into Clinical Practice*. London: Routledge, Taylor & Francis Group.

Morrison, M.D. & Rammage, L.A. (1993). Muscle misuse voice disorders: Description and classification. *Acta Otolaryngology*, 113, 3, 428–434.

O'Brian, S., Packman, A. & Onslow, M. (2010). The Camperdown program. In B. Guitar & R. McCauley (eds.), *Treatment of Stuttering: Established and Emerging Interventions*. Philadelphia, PA: Wolters Kluwer/Lippincott Williams & Wilkins.

Poburka, B. (2002). Voice and stuttering therapy: Finding common ground. www.mnsu.edu/comdis/isad5/papers/poburka.html [Accessed February 2021].

Runyan, C.M. & Runyan, S. (1993). Therapy for school-age stutterers: An update on the fluency rules program. In R. Curlee (ed.), *Stuttering and Related Disorders of Fluency*. New York: Thieme Medical Publishers Inc.

Shapiro, D. (1999). *Stuttering Intervention*. Austin, TX: ProEd.

Shine, R.E. (1988). *Systematic Fluency Training for Young Children*, 3rd edition. Austin, TX: ProEd.

Turnbull, J. & Stewart, T. (2017). *The Dysfluency Resource Book*, 2nd edition. London: Routledge, Taylor & Francis Group.

Weiner, A.E. (1984). Vocal control therapy for stutterers. In M. Peins (ed.), *Contemporary Approaches in Stuttering Therapy*. Boston: Little, Brown & Company.

Williams, D. & Brutten, G. (1994). Physiologic and aerodynamic events prior to the speech of stutterers and nonstutterers. *Journal of Fluency Disorders*, 19, 2, 83–111.

Section G

THERAPY

Stammering modification or 'stammer more easily' approach

60. WHAT IS THE STAMMERING MODIFICATION APPROACH?

Stammer more easily or stammering modification is based on the idea that a large part of stammering consists of what the person does to avoid stammering: his struggle, fear, tension-filled behaviours and avoidance of the 'core' of stammering. Various techniques are introduced by the therapist to facilitate changing the person's stammer from one which encompasses tension and struggle to one that does not.

The approach usually starts with assertiveness training and desensitisation. (See **Section E, Points 47 and 49.**) This is followed by intervention which focuses on processes which modify the overt features of stammering to the extent that they become more relaxed and less impactful on the individual's communication. Unlike fluency-enhancing techniques, the whole of the PWS's speech delivery does not require change, only the moments of dysfluency. As Shapiro (1999) describes (referencing Guitar & Peters 1980):

> "stuttering modification is a dynamic process in which the PWS is not directed to speak in an abnormal pattern (as in fluency shaping) but is expected and supported to confront his communication-related fears and avoidances (unlike fluency shaping)."
>
> (p. 189)

The aim of a stammering modification approach is not to produce fluent speech as an end product, although a client might find that his fluency does increase. Rather, the objective is for the PWS to gradually reduce the tense and out-of-control forms of dysfluency, changing these to behaviours which are less effortful and smoother. In doing so, the PWS will also indirectly address some of his negative feelings and attitudes to stammering. The revised pattern of talking is less debilitating than the tense, out-of-control forms of dysfluency which it replaces: a gentler form of stammering.

In this approach, there are none of the delineated, hierarchical, linguistic frames of the fluency-shaping approach, no GILCU-based exercises. Instead, the key to the approach is an unstructured but careful conversation and problem-solving dialogue between the PWS and his clinician. The overall rate of change can be slower than other approaches, but the PWS is an active participant in the process rather than one following instructions. The therapist requires particular skills to engage the PWS, which Shapiro (1999) states include:

> "providing emotional support, clinical problem solving, and responding to client's individual differences."
>
> (p. 189)

As such, it may be more difficult for a newly qualified or beginning specialist SLT to undertake. Learning from theoretical-based instructions can be problematic, so the recommended route to become competent in stammering modification is to watch a more experienced or specialist colleague engaging directly with a client. In the absence of a specialist SLT who can act as a mentor, there are videos/DVDs available from the British Stammering Association and Stuttering Foundation of America and some on YouTube. (The recordings of Van Riper working with an adult are decades old but are nevertheless worthwhile viewing.) Although it may be difficult, new clinicians should not be put off learning how to implement this approach, as it is an important option to offer to a PWS.

61. BACKGROUND

Van Riper (1973), the father of stammering modification techniques, based his approach on three theories:

1. learning theory; the PWS learns how to unlearn his dysfluent behaviours and replace them with easier, less disruptive ones
2. servotheory; Van Riper believed that stammering was connected to disruptions in auditory processing. Consequently, he stressed the need for the client to monitor his speech using a variety of means (such as proprioception, visual and kinaesthetic senses) rather than purely auditory feedback
3. psychotherapy; acknowledging the negative thoughts and emotions associated with stammering, Van Riper recognised the need for interventions to manage these issues in addition to direct speech work.

Based on his studies of stammering, Van Riper (1973) concluded that a PWS anticipated dysfluency and therefore formed what he called 'preparatory sets'. Once this was initiated, the person went on to stammer in the way he had predicted. Thus, in stammering modification therapy, the individual learns not to anticipate but to adopt a new way of setting his motor speech system to counter his old speech pattern. As Manning (2001) notes, this is quite a challenging task:

> "Changing the well-practiced and stable patterns of these surface features of stuttering is no easy process. The old patterns are not only well-learned, they are comfortable. The new, better ways of speaking will feel awkward and strange, at least until they are practiced enough to become habituated."
>
> (p. 284)

62. WITH WHOM TO USE STAMMERING MODIFICATION?

Due to the complexity of the process, it is recommended that it be used with older teenagers and adults. However, the severity of the stammer which a PWS has should not be a factor when deciding whether to offer it as a therapy option. According to Guitar and Peters (1980):

> "This approach works as well with mild as with severe stutterers. The important thing to consider is how much the stutterer avoids or hides his stuttering. If he spends considerable energy disguising his stuttering, he is more likely to profit from stuttering modification therapy."
>
> (p. 34)

Shapiro (1999) lists a number of observable features which would indicate the approach is appropriate for an individual:

- hides or disguises his stuttering
- avoids speaking
- perceives personal penalty as a consequence of stuttering
- feels poorly about himself as a communicator
- demonstrates a more positive response to stuttering modification trial (i.e. is able to discuss the nature of observed fluency and stammering, practice different ways of stammering, talk about feelings and attitudes about himself as a communicator.)

(p. 192)

Turnbull and Stewart (2017), when talking specifically about the use of block modification (see **Point 66**), have slightly different indicators for a client:

- must have closely identified what it is he does when he stammers
- be sufficiently desensitised to his stammering
- have a sufficient number of at least moderately severe blocks
- [In the case of a person who back-tracks, i.e. someone approaches a difficult word and then goes

back and repeats one or more words as a run-in]
the person should be helped to 'move forward' in
his speech before learning block modification
- needs to have had some experimentation with
change, both in non-speech and speech.

(p. 179)

Note: This is a slightly different view from what I am now advocating. In the therapy section, I recommend the use of openness, desensitisation, voluntary stammering and avoidance reduction as relevant introductory interventions to be considered for many, if not all, approaches and not solely for stammering modification. (See **Section E, Points 48–51**.)

63. HOW TO TEACH STAMMERING MODIFICATION

The stages, according to Van Riper (1973), are:

- identification
- desensitisation
- variation
- modification
- stabilisation.

Each one of these stages will be described in detail in the following sections, with the exception of desensitisation, which can be found as one of the common interventions (see **Point 49**), and stabilisation, which will be discussed as part of relapse planning (see **Section J**).

64. IDENTIFICATION

Van Riper (1973) discusses the importance of this phase of the process. He lists a number of reasons why it is necessary to begin with identification. In his view, identification:

- sets the collaborative agenda for the client-clinician relationship
- specifies the problem in terms of what needs to be unlearned

- places the responsibility for change on the shoulders of the PWS
- sets out the analytic approach that is needed
- uses examples from outside as well as within clinic and so helps the process of generalisation
- does not require immediate modification of the stammer, which could be too difficult for the client at this stage
- shows the client that the therapist is accepting of his stammer and is not judgmental
- contributes to desensitisation.

During the process of assessment, the PWS and clinician will have been involved in identifying the make-up of the person's stammer. Both the overt features (i.e. above the iceberg's water line) and those below the surface (i.e. the covert features) will have been scrutinised. While identification, as the initial part of a stammering modification approach, has some similarities to the previous assessment, there are additional features which make it a more in-depth and challenging process.

For example, in the initial assessment, the PWS may have been asked to differentiate the observable features of his stammer; pick out repetitions, prolongations, avoidances and so on. In the identification phase of stammering modification, he is asked to go further and pinpoint more precisely and in depth those behaviours that occur:

- before a stammering event
- during the stammering itself
- after the stammering has ended.

Ross attended group therapy sessions when in his early twenties. His stammer was characterised by marked silent and audible blocks with significant laryngeal and oral tension. He was frustrated and angry with his stammer and would often stop mid-stammer to swear or bang furniture in his distress. His identification based on this sequential approach would look like this:

> Before stammering: increased heart rate, faster breathing, churning feelings in stomach, tightening diaphragm,

thinking about problematic word, looking for other words that I could substitute, looking at the immediate environment for who might hear my stammer, looking away from listener.

During stammer: breath held, throat locked, no sound, diaphragm rigid, jaw moving up and down (feels out of control) eyes closed, tapping foot or toes in my shoes, shoulders lifted, inward focus on stammer, (black in front of my eyes), thoughts of 'when will this end?', 'it's going on forever', 'I can't breathe', 'will I pass out?', panic.

After stammer: rapid breathing, feelings of release, but remaining tension in jaw and shoulders, have to actively put my shoulders down to release the tension, eyes open but unable to look at listener, dare not look beyond myself to others around me or my listener, dread their reactions, angry at myself and my stammer, frustrated at why this happens to me, I finish off what I have to say as quickly as possible, have thoughts of how I can get out of the rest of the conversation and leave the situation as quickly as possible.

Summary of Ross's Identification Chart

	Before stammer	During stammer	After stammer
Anxiety	Increased heart rate	Breath held	Rapid breathing
	Increase in breathing rate		
	Churning in stomach		
Tension	Diaphragm	Diaphragm	Jaw
		Throat	Shoulders
		Shoulders	

(Continued)

(*Continued*)

	Before stammer	During stammer	After stammer
Thoughts	About the specific word	'When will this end?'	'How can I end this conversation?'
	Thinking of possible alternative words	'It's going on forever.'	'I need to get away.'
		'I can't breathe.'	
		'Will I pass out?'	
Awareness and feelings	Concern about who is going to hear me stammer	Panic	Release
			Dread (of others negative reactions)
			Anger (bang table)
			Frustration, shame
Eye contact and focus	Look away from listener/communication partner	Eyes closed	Eyes open (but unable to look at listener)
		Inward focus	Inward focus
		Black in front of my eyes	Unable to look around
Speech		No sound	Rapid speech on rest of sentence
		Jaw moving up and down	

	Before stammer	During stammer	After stammer
		Feeling out of control	
		Swearing	

By setting it out in this way, the therapist can address any gaps in his observation. For example, in this instance, there appears to be no consideration of his speech prior to the onset of stammering. It suggests a block modification approach, especially the pre-block phase, would be useful to him, for example, using some positive preparation such as relaxed articulation might help. In addition, his inward focus during and after his stammer is preventing him from checking the validity of his pre-emptions about his communication partner and others around him reacting negatively to his dysfluency.

This exercise allows an overview of the stammer; identification can then proceed to unpick the issues in more detail.

Difficulties: When asked to describe his stammer, a PWS will often struggle. He may lump together the myriad of behaviours that make up his dysfluency into one 'stammering' label and have difficulty separating them all out. Alternatively, he can focus on one single aspect of his stammer, the feature that he is most concerned with or is aware of or that has been noticed and commented on by others (e.g. multiple repetitions, jaw jerking, tongue protrusion). Consequently, one of the aims of identification is to pull the stammer apart into its various components, and in this way, it is easier to manage. A further aim of this stage of the 'stammer more easily' approach is to enable the individual to become aware of the great variety of stammers he has, from minor hesitations which occur in everyone's speech to other more intrusive patterns such as longer vowel prolongations and finally the marked dysfluencies that disrupt and evoke a significant emotional response.

Emotional response: Throughout this process, the therapist needs to be aware of the impact this work will have on the PWS. It will be difficult for him to engage with, as she will be asking him to look in the face of his dysfluency, something which he has probably avoided doing for a long time. He will need understanding and support in the discrimination of the components of stammering. In addition, he is likely to experience some emotional response such as anger, denial, shame or fear when coming face to face with his stammer. Consequently, the clinician needs to proceed cautiously and with great sensitivity, checking frequently with the individual in front of her that he is coping with the process.

> "Since our aim is also to reduce the attendant emotionality, the analytical examination of the displayed behavior in the context of the therapist's genuine interest and freedom from punitiveness reduces anxiety."
>
> (Van Riper 1973, p. 247)

Identification hierarchy: Van Riper (1973) recommends an hierarchy of the processes of identification in therapy. In order:

i.   a PWS is asked to identify episodes of fluency. The amount of fluent speech he has already may surprise a client, as his focus is on the dysfluent aspect of his talking.
ii. then he is required to gather examples of short, easy stammers or, as Van Riper calls them, 'the fluent stutterings'. This task in particular illustrates to the PWS that there are many different ways of stammering, which he had perhaps been unaware of. These smaller, 'more fluent' versions he might find easier to live alongside but also show him what his target is and that it is already a part of his speaking, at the very beginning of the process.
iii. there is an exploration of the smaller, subtle changes that a PWS often carries out in order to put off saying, or prepare to say, the problematic word or sound; his 'preparatory set'. For example, changing word order, taking a deep breath prior to the word which he might not need, increasing the tension in his articulators and so on. This is often accompanied by significant negative feelings, which should also be explored in a gentle manner.

iv. it is recommended that an individual and his therapist explore his speech in clinic, perhaps recording examples and looking at them/playing them back, sharing what they have seen and heard together. Later the client can look for examples in other settings with the support of a significant other who has been briefed beforehand on what is required.
v. finally, we turn to identifying the core of stammering.

(Note: Van Riper [1973] works on identifying avoidance behaviours at this point. But in the approach I am advocating, the avoidance work has already been carried out at a much earlier stage, making the stammering more overt and easier to access and change.)

In this phase, Van Riper (1973) talks about a system of comparison between a triad or three examples of the person's speech: the core or what he calls 'abnormal' utterance, the 'fluent stammers' and the 'normal' utterance. In this 'compare and contrast' exercise, the individual is invited to explore how they are each physically produced: the behaviours that define each of the examples.

> "we are seeking to alter the stutterer's usual bias toward monitoring his speech acoustically rather than proprioceptively. We want him to stop listening to the gaps and abnormal sounds in his speech and to start finding out what he is actually doing."
>
> (p. 257)

It is recommended that a therapist and PWS start identifying the differences that are visible before moving on the kinaesthetic, visual and acoustic distinctions. 'Saying the word "so", how did you place your mouth when it was easy to say? And look at your lip position. What is happening there? Are you anticipating the /s/ or some other sound?' This way of looking directly at core stammering in a pseudo-scientific way allows the individual to take a step back and be a more objective listener/observer. However, the clinician needs to be alert to the possibility that the activity will be challenging for the individual and that it often raises emotional issues for him.

In this process, a PWS often wants to experiment with changing his production. However, this is not the aim of this stage of modification; that comes later. Nevertheless, if an individual wants to experiment with the difference at this point, then it reflects well on his engagement in the exercise and his motivation for change.

Specific areas of attention: There are a couple of specific areas that Van Riper (1973) recommends the PWS focus on during this identification process. First, identifying the 'loci of tension', that is, particular areas of muscle tightening and strain associated with the production of specific sounds. Second, what he calls the identification of 'repetitive recoil behaviors'. In this latter exercise, the PWS is asked to explore those repetitions or oscillations which appear to be 'run ins' or making an attempt at a sound/word and then pulling back from it. These are different from repetitions of the same sounds often heard as part of stammering. The difference is that these attempts are not related to the target phoneme. For example, when trying to say 'see' /si/, the person may repeat the word with additional starter words or phrases, such as 'well, /sə sə sə/ well /sə sə sə/'. Having the PWS identify that his repetitions are unrelated to the sound or word he is trying to say can be an important realisation and one which is a first stage in inhibiting this particular issue.

65. VARIATION

As part of the 'pre requisite skills' outlined in preparing for change (see **Section E, Point 47**), an individual will have carried out a number of variation tasks in relation to non-speech behaviour, such as changing the route he takes to work, what he eats for lunch, where he buys his groceries and so on. In this section, the focus is on variation of speech-related behaviours.

Speech variation. This is a good place to start when looking to change a person's speaking pattern. There are features of speech which are more easily modified:

- volume, that is, slightly louder or quieter voice production. This can be altered in relation to whom the person is speaking, choosing a specific situation to use a certain volume and/or a change across a sentence (e.g. increasing or decreasing volume as the sentence ends)

- speed, that is, an increase or decrease of speaking rate. Experiments can be done again in relation to a communication partner, a specific situation and/or across the length of a sentence
- intonation and stress patterns, that is, increasing or decreasing the amount of melody in speech. Variations would include making the stress patterns more regular; creating a flatter, less interesting production; or the alternative – a highly varied voice production with a greater range of intonation and stressed syllables.

Stammering variation. The objective of this work is to diminish the strength of particular behaviours by altering them in some way. There are a number of ways this can be achieved (which can be enhanced by the use of video/video playback, if available):

> Learn to vary the stammering is really important before you try stutter modification.
> Kato Polfliet (Personal Communication 2021)

- disrupting the postponements or run-ins. This can be done by altering the specific, habitual run-in. For example, Linda used 'You know' before a problematic word. She was invited to think of a number of alternatives she could use and identified 'I know', 'we know' and 'well' as options. It was useful that she was able to select from three other possibilities rather than just substituting one for another.

  Another disrupting variation behaviour is to double the run-in; so, in Linda's example, she would say 'You know, you know'. A PWS is often sceptical about the validity of such an option, but in my experience, it is an extremely disruptive possibility which has a significant and often immediate impact.
- a clinician might also suggest that the person try and reduce and ultimately remove the run-ins altogether. This can be

achieved by focusing on moving forward in speech and resisting the temptation to go back over something that has already been said. Such an exercise depends on the PWS being able to concentrate on his production and monitor the occurrence of postponements. This is only manageable in some situations, which should be discussed and determined with the individual.

- changing a sequence of behaviour. Detailed identification will have shown how an individual orders his stammering. Disrupting the sequence will diminish the strength of the behaviour. So, if Ollie closes his eyes first, followed by increasing the tension in his lips, he will be invited to tighten his lips first, keeping his eyes open and only closing them once the lip posture has been achieved.

- varying in the moment of stammering. In this exercise, the clinician stammers alongside the PWS, following precisely the pattern of his behaviour. She then models a slightly different movement, and the individual is asked to vary his stammer in the moment by following her change. It is important that the therapist know the person's stammer almost as well as he knows it himself if this procedure is to be successful. In addition, the PWS and clinician must be fully synchronised, observing closely their stammering behaviours and the modifications that are being made.

At the end of this phase, as Van Riper (1973) describes:

> "The stutterer has now learned to identify his various stuttering behaviors; he has become desensitized, at least to some degree, . . . and he has found that he can alter and vary his stuttering reactions and himself."
>
> (p. 311)

It is now time to move onto the next stage: modification.

66. BLOCK MODIFICATION

This is an interesting technique for a PWS for many reasons. First, he works 'backwards', that is, working from *after* the block, then *in* the block and last *before* the block. In order to do this, it is crucial that he be able to concentrate on moving forward through the dysfluency and eliminating his backtracking or postponements. If he does not do this, then the technique will not be effective.

Second, it is a highly rewarding competence, as the person does not fail. After he has learnt all the possible ways he can modify his block, he has options; if he misses the pre-block phase, he has the opportunity to 'catch' the stammer during its occurrence (in-block); if that goes by, then he is still able to make some response after the block has ended (post-block).

It can be a complicated process to explain, and I recommend using a visual representation in the first instance to help the PWS see an overview more easily. There is a simple diagram in Turnbull and Stewart (2017) which may be used to introduce block modification in its entirety. After this introduction, the technique is then worked on by breaking it down into three parts: post-block, in-block and pre-block modification.

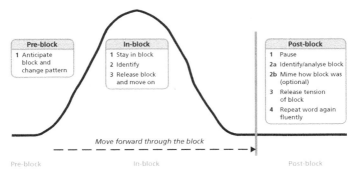

Figure 7.1 A Visual Representation of the Stages of Block Modification

i. Post-block modification (or cancellation Van Riper 1973). This is probably the most important phase of block modification and one whose implementation should not be rushed. It provides the foundation on which all the other phases are based. It consists of a number of parts: pause, reduplication and then production of the target word.

- The pause. First, the person finishes the block and immediately introduces a pause into his talking before continuing on with the rest of his utterance. The effect of
  the pause, according to Van Riper, is to make a definite
  separation between the dysfluency and the speech which
  follows, which is very likely to be fluent. In this way,
  the dysfluent speech is not 'rewarded' with a period of
  fluency. The length of the pause is important. It should
  be long enough for the individual to register the ending
  of his block and to enable him to carry out some activities (which will come later) within this created space.
  Van Riper suggests a pause that lasts long enough for
  the person to say 'hippopotamus' internally/silently
  three times, that is, equivalent to about three seconds.

  Turnbull and Stewart (2017) recommend the pause
  be used on the severest blocks in the first instance, and
  then when the PWS is proficient with this, he can move
  to applying pauses to less severe blocks.

  Difficulties that may arise: an individual can struggle
  to pause immediately after his block. It may be a couple
  of words later before he realises the block has occurred
  and he is able to stop. This is a scenario that can be rec-
  tified easily; given time and attention, the person can
  bring his focus to the block earlier and earlier and will
  be able to stop immediately after the block.

  Giving the pause sufficient time may also be problematic. He will rush the pause if he still equates silence
  with blocking and finds it difficult to sit with quiet as
  a result. If this is the case, then further work on tolerating silence may be necessary before work on this
  stage of block modification can continue. (See **Section E,
  Point 49**.)

  Once pausing is a regular feature after blocking,
  the individual can move to using the pause for two
  activities. First, he uses the pause to be calm and relax
  areas of tension he identifies in his body and/or speech
  musculature. Employing two or three diaphragmatic
  breaths is helpful here. Second, when he is sufficiently

composed, he can employ the pause as time to identify the features of the stammer that have just occurred. Using proprioceptive, visual, kinaesthetic and auditory awareness, he should notice:

- ◦ the position of his articulators
- ◦ areas of tension
- ◦ eye closure
- ◦ sounds he makes
- ◦ any accessory movements.

- • Reduplication. The next step is often very challenging for a PWS, as it involves him confronting the core of his stammering. He is now required, within the pause, to reproduce, in mime, a shortened version of his stammer. This is followed immediately by a modified version of the same behaviour: a struggle-free, easier version of the same word. There will be times when the person cannot do this step due to the communication context, so outside practice needs to be realistically tailored to his situation, for example, limiting the mime and repetition to his home/family setting and/or conversations with a well-briefed SO.

- • Repeat the target word fluently. Finally, the mime is dropped and the individual says the word again, having internalised what he needs to do in order to achieve an easier version of the same word. Van Riper (1973) states that this repetition should be spoken 'slower, stronger' and 'more carefully and consciously', and in so doing, he makes the listener aware that he has recognised a difference in his speech and is doing something to change it. It is important that the PWS does not rush away from the moment of stammering. In other words, this stage of repeating the target word is done with conscious awareness, setting up the next part of the person's utterance with minimal tension and urgency.

Note: A PWS may find that this stage is sufficient for him to manage his blocks, but other individuals will continue through the programme to learn the remaining two modifications (in-block and pre-block) and then have options when and how to handle their dysfluencies.

Summary of post block modification.

1. Complete the block
2. Complete the block and pause immediately after
3. Complete the block, pause and be calm,
4. Complete the block, pause, be calm, identify areas of tension
5. Complete the block, pause, be calm and mime how the block occurred
6. Complete the block, pause, be calm, mime block and mime an easier production of the word (eliminating the blocking behaviours)
7. Complete the block, pause, be calm, and repeat target word in struggle-free, easier way.

ii. In-block modification (or pull-outs Van Riper 1973). In this stage, the PWS takes control of the moment of his stammering and modifies his behaviour as it is happening. Van Riper notes that a client often moves from post-block cancellation into this stage automatically:

> "The modifications of behavior learned through cancellation tend to move forward in time to manifest themselves during the period of stuttering itself."
>
> (p. 328)

At the start, an individual is rewarded for any attempt he makes to 'get hold' of his stammer as it happens: letting go of tension, slowing down the articulation. Whenever he has made a positive attempt at pulling out of his stammer, then he does not need to cancel the word and proceeds with the rest of his sentence. In this way, his effort is rewarded.

As work proceeds, the therapist will help the person become more proficient at changing his behaviour as it happens. She will direct him to specific, more effective changes based on what she is observing him do. For example: Djo, in saying the word 'where', pushed his lips forward, increasing the tension in his jaw; closed his eyes; and lengthened the sound. The therapist encouraged him to stay with the stammer and pull his jaw back, releasing the tension, then worked on changing the lip posture to a gentler /w/ before getting him to open his eyes.

It is crucial that the PWS not stop and try to say the word again. The principal of always moving forward during stammering is played out in this in-block modification as in the previous phase.

Other Examples of In-block Modifications

In-block modifications	
Types of stammering	Therapist directions
Blocking on /k/ of 'can'	
Tongue pushed against alveolar ridge	Release tension in tongue
Jaw tight	Open jaw slightly
Larynx locked	Allow air flow over cords
Silent block on /o/ of orange	
Larynx locked	Use vocal fry to initiate phonation. Then change to normal phonation. Continue to produce a prolonged vowel
Tongue lifted	Lower tongue tip to relaxed position
Mouth fully open	Slightly reduce degree of mouth opening

The way in which the therapist directs the person is by offering modifications for him to try out and see which works. It does not matter in which order she offers her ideas. The principle is one of experimenting to see what works. In this same spirit of experimentation, she can model the change behaviours alongside her client in the moment of his stammer, providing him with a visual and auditory representation of changes he could make. As this process progresses, the PWS comes to realise which modifications work best for the specific behaviours he has. In this way, altering his stammer in the moment becomes easier and less random.

If the person is unable to modify a moment of stammering, then he always has the 'safety net' of a post-block technique, and in this way, the dysfluency does not progress unmodified.

iii. Pre-block modification. This final step aims to modify the anticipation of stammering or the initiation of 'preparatory sets' (as mentioned previously in **Point 64** of this section). Once again, it is often the case that a client will move to this phase without being instructed to do so. He has learned to manage his behaviours within a block and is able to apply this learning to the point where he prepares to say problematic sounds. His pre-planning in this instance is not the old 'preparatory set' for stammering but the newly learnt smoothing out of stammering he has rehearsed in both in-block and post-block modification.

When approaching a word he anticipates stammering on, the PWS pauses, relaxes his speech musculature and moment-arily plans how to say the word, learning from his previous experiments. For example, he may use light articulatory contact, as he knows from his experience that he tends to tighten his tongue and lips, or he may take a calm breath rather than taking in too much air, which creates too much air pressure for his vocal cords to manage.

Again, he can use in block or cancellation if his pre-set is not successful; thus, he is always working positively on his speech.

Summary of Stammering Modification Techniques: Everard, R.A. & Howell, P. (2018) report on a stammering modification approach from the user's perspective. There is also a video summarising all the processes involved in block modification available on Vimeo: https://vimeo.com/553899193, *Explaining Block Modification: A Tutorial by Dr Trudy Stewart.*

In addition, the following chart provides an example around the production of /s/ of the word stammer, which may be helpful for a client to see.

Client using modification techniques on /s/ of the word 'stammer'		
Pre-block modification	In-block modification	Post-block modification
Anticipates old 'pre-paratory set'	x	x
Relaxes articulators	x	x
Uses diaphragmatic breathing	x	x
x	Continues to pro-long /s/	x
x	Gradually lessens tension in articulators	x
x	Eases out of /s/ and onto /t/ and then into vowel	x
x	x	Finishes block
x	x	Pauses (during pauses, calms, releases tension, identifies stammering pattern)
x	x	Repeats target word without struggle

(Continued)

(*Continued*)

Client using modification techniques on /s/ of the word 'stammer'		
Pre-block modification	In-block modification	Post-block modification
x	x	Continues with rest of sentence in slow, calm way (i.e. not rushing away from dysfluency)

REFERENCES

Everard, R.A. & Howell, P. (2018). We have a voice: Exploring participants' experiences of stuttering modification therapy. *American Journal of Speech & Language Pathology, 27,* 3S, 273–1286.

Guitar, B. & Peters, T.J. (1980). *Stuttering: An Integration of Contemporary Therapies.* Memphis: TN: Stuttering Foundation of America.

Manning, W.H. (2001). *Clinical Decision Making in Fluency Disorders.* Canada: Singular Thompson Learning.

Shapiro, D. (1999). *Stuttering Intervention.* Austin, TX: ProEd.

Turnbull, J. & Stewart, T. (2017). *The Dysfluency Resource Book,* 2nd edition. London: Routledge, Taylor & Francis Group.

Van Riper, C. (1973). *The Treatment of Stuttering.* Englewood Cliffs, NJ: Prentice-Hall, Inc.

OTHER RESOURCES

Cheasman, C., Everard, R. & Simpson, S. (2013). *Stammering from the Inside: New Perspectives on Working with Young People and Adults.* Havant: J.R. Press.

Van Riper, C. *Adult Stuttering Therapy.* This single DVD, over six hours long, reproduces all of Van Riper's classic series of nine videotapes on this subject. They depict the management of stammering from the evaluation interview, through seven therapy sessions, to both 1-year and 20-year follow-up. Available from the British Stammering Association/ Stamma and Stuttering Foundation of America.

Section H

THERAPY
'Stammer more proudly'

67. OPENING COMMENTS

There appears to be a growing interest in the views of those who subscribe to a way of thinking about stammering that has been called 'stammer more proudly' (Simpson et al. 2021). In this section, I will describe the genesis of this new set of beliefs and its aims for a PWS. I hope to provide particular points of relevance for newly qualified therapists so they can support any PWS in making an informed choice around which therapy option he may wish to pursue. I will draw heavily on the writings, including personal blogs, and conversations I have had with many individuals who support the 'stammer more proudly' movement, including Patrick Campbell, Sam Simpson, Katy Bailey, Kath Bond, SLTs in the Yorkshire CEN and others and members of the Doncaster self-help group. While I have included some SLT comments, it is important that the voice of the PWS be the most authoritative in this section.

68. WHAT IS 'STAMMERING PRIDE?'

Here are the views of a number of PWS from the Doncaster self-help group. When asked what 'stammering pride' meant to them, they said:

> "What comes to my mind when I hear 'stammering pride' is: to embrace, to accept, and to make stammering visible. Stammering pride is the opposite of the feelings of shame most of us experience at certain points in our lives when fighting too hard to hide

 DOI: 10.4324/9781003177890-9

or 'cure' something that is just a characteristic of our speech."

"Stammering pride: Owning one's own stammering. Viewing it just as 'the way we talk' due to brain difference. The problem isn't mine, because I stammer, it's a societal issue. Much like society excluding wheelchair users by not providing ramps. The media have a lot to answer for! Being open and speaking about stammering helps others to understand it, which in turn engenders change—albeit slowly!"

69. THE SOCIAL MODEL OF DISABILITY

Much of current understanding and management of stammering is largely based on a medical model which views disability as a 'problem' that belongs to the disabled individual; a client attends a clinic, often in a medical setting, and is assessed by an expert, who confirms a diagnosis and directs a management plan. In this scenario, the PWS is a recipient of therapy that is often 'instructional' and may have a manual for the clinician to follow.

(Note: Much of this book steers away from the medical model, illustrating a collaborative way of working in which the therapist and PWS jointly determine a tailor-made, individualised plan and experiment in a therapeutic process. See **Section E, Point 46**.)

The 'stammer more proudly' approach is based on principles that differ from the medical model. Campbell (2018) wrote:

"The exact definition remains abstract to us, it is a variable mish-mash of ideologies, drawing from the social model, political model, neurodiversity movement and, more generally, a socially progressive cultural backdrop."

www.redefiningstammering.co.uk/fresh-eyes/

Let us consider first the influence of the social model of disability. This model, described by Oliver (1990) (drawing on the work of Hunt 1966), differentiates between disability and impairment. A person may have an impairment, such as deafness or mental illness, but this may or may not be a disability. The degree of disability experienced by the individual is determined by the barriers, stigma or prejudices which exist in society. For example, a man who has limited vision is not disabled in his home, where he has access to well-lit areas, flooring which defines the demarcation of different rooms, reading items written in Braille and so on. However, when he steps into a local cafe, which has poor lighting, lack of space between tables and no menus written in Braille, he is unable to function in an independent way and will require assistance to be seated and make a choice of beverage. The cafe, due to its inaccessibility for people of different visual abilities, has turned his impairment into a disability.

70. SOCIAL MODEL AND STAMMERING

A person has an observable stammer which he experiences in most speaking situations. However, his mode of communication becomes a disability when he is required to use voice recognition devices and when other people do not wait for him to complete his sentences or treat him as if he were of inferior intellect. Similarly, a person with an interiorised stammer will be disabled in situations where he is required to say specific words or phrases and given no choice, such as having to give personal details or answering forced alternative questions.

71. CRITICAL THEORY

The second model which has relevance to 'stammer more proudly' thinking is critical theory. Such a theory aims to reveal to an individual the form of social or other oppression that he is experiencing by visible or invisible systems (e.g. racism, sexism) exercised by dominant groups. It seeks to explain what is wrong and detail the alteration which is needed. The objective is to free the person from specific oppression and to achieve some societal change. One such form of oppression relevant to stammering is 'ableism': the way society is organised in favour of able-bodied individuals and the fluent or 'able-speaking'.

72. CRITICAL THEORY AND STAMMERING

Society values fluent speech; fluent speakers are the prominent voices in the world, selected to be heard in the media and elsewhere (Claypole 2021). Those individuals with different levels of fluency are rarely heard, and when they are, for example, in film and dramas, it is often a stereotyped depiction, such as a person with underlying psychological traits and vulnerability or someone lacking intelligence, being weak, anxious or nervous (Johnson 2008).

73. THE THERAPY CONTEXT

Stewart (1995) expressed concern that the management of stammering by SLTs was creating 'square pegs', that is, individuals who could neither engage on the same terms in the fluent world nor be true to their stammering selves in the environment in which they lived and worked.

> "we [SLTs] teach clients to speak more fluently, rarely with a naturalness accepted as the norm by others or facilitate clients to accept their stammer while perhaps lessening its severity and impact on their lives. But the fact remains that they stammer in a society whose view of stammerers is still that of nervous, anxious stereotypes."
>
> (p. 482)

Stewart went on to argue for SLTs to embrace an educative role and help a generation accept dysfluent speech: 'in the same way as society has come to accept the notion of disability' (p. 482).

In the same paper, a PWS wrote of the paradox he experienced in the therapy process of being more open and accepting of his stammer:

"The outside world pats me on the back when I don't stammer and there's part of me that agrees with them. They tell me how impressed they are with my progress and it reinforces the idea of suppressing my stammer and hiding it, something that I used to do all the time before I entered into therapy. It would seem that I can change myself but I can't change the world."

(Daly in Stewart 1995, p. 482)

In a similar vein, Campbell (2019a) has written of his understanding of his stammer in terms of the societal oppression:

"I now realise my desire for fluency reflects the pervasive stigma and discrimination towards stammering in our society, which has ultimately come to reside in me as self-stigma and oppression of my own stammering."

Stamma website [accessed March 2021]

74. MOBILISATION OF THE STAMMERING COMMUNITY

Since Stewart's paper, some SLTs have been engaged in lobbying for individuals who stammer, but more importantly, those who stammer have become active in speaking out for themselves and arguing that their voices be heard. For example, in the United States, a blog, *Did I Stutter*, and a podcast, *StutterTalk*, have been influential in raising the profile of stammer pride. Here in the United Kingdom, those who advocate 'stammer more proudly' are an important part of this mobilisation and play a key role, in critical theory terms, in bringing oppression to the fore, specifying what is wrong and what needs to change.

> Being fluent or non-fluent does not make us a better or a worse person.
> No one has chosen to stutter. For this reason SLTs and others should try to create such conditions for acceptance in order for PWS to be fully accepted in society.
> Jan Dezort (Personal Communication 2021)

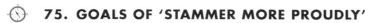

75. GOALS OF 'STAMMER MORE PROUDLY'

In a recent paper at the Oxford Dysfluency Conference, Simpson et al. (2021) put forward their non-medicalised, working definition of stammering:

> "Stammering is a neuro-developmental variation that leads to an unpredictable and unique forward execution of speech sounds produced in the context of language and social interaction."

They also outlined the goals of the 'stammer more proudly' movement. I will list them here and reference in more detail some of the writing and research around the individual points where possible.

> The acceptance of neurodiversity. There is evidence to suggest stammering has a neurological basis in many individuals. Rather than regard this evidence as a pathology, it can be viewed as part of the neurological diversity of speaking rather than something abnormal. Just as there are many ways of walking, there is a wide variety of types of talking. Some of these modes include voices which are higher pitched, more hoarse, louder, less fast and less fluent. This does not make dysfluency (or indeed any of the other variations) less acceptable or invalid, just different. The 'stammer more proudly' movement is keen that stammering be seen and accepted by society in this way.

> "Dysfluent speech expresses a difference, not a deviance, and re-defining stuttering in non-medicalized terms is essential for stuttering activism to carve a place for dysfluent voices in the world."
>
> (Pierre 2019, p. 13)

Watch your language! 'Stammering more proudly' has challenged the stammering community and those affiliated with it to consider the messages conveyed to others by the language which is employed. The language commonly used around stammering frequently has negative connotations, such as an individual being 'afflicted by' or 'handicapped by' stammering. Similarly, a PWS is described as 'struggling to overcome' his stammer, as if he were waging a war against an arch-enemy.

The writer David Mitchell, a PWS himself, makes a similar robust and frank point in a lecture given in Holland in 2016 called 'Thirteen Ways of Looking at a Stammer'. In point 11, entitled: 'A Stammer Is Not an Enemy, but a Part of Yourself', he said:

> "I view phrases such as 'overcoming your stammer' or 'conquering your disfluency' with suspicion – such language comes from the same ignorant and/ or cruel mindset that says we lack will-power. The military metaphor turns stammerers into perpetual losers in a battle which we're too crap ever to win."
>
> (p. 8)

All of us, that is, SLTs, educators, authors, family members and sometimes those who stammer, must be mindful of how we talk and write about stammering. Albeit unconsciously, at times, we can contribute to the narrative that 'stammering is bad and fluency is better'. This undermines stammering, ignores the part it plays in the diversity of speaking and invalidates the contribution those who stammer are able to gift to society. Cole (2020), in an article on the Stamma (British Stammering Association) website, wrote:

> "what we must do as adults is to look to find better ways of reacting to individuals stumbling on their words and change the language that we use to address it. Be it a teacher imploring a student to 'slow down and take their time' or a manager telling a colleague to 'calm down and breathe', even if they are intended to be helpful, these phrases only serve to heighten tension and cultivate a

negative mindset towards public speaking and to
stammering itself."
    Stamma website [accessed April 2021] (Cole 2020)

In October 2020, the BSA launched a campaign called 'Find
the Right Words' which demonstrated how to change the
language and perception of stammering.

> "'Find the Right Words' aims to kick-start a con-
> versation around the negative language used when
> talking about stammering, and help those who
> don't stammer to understand that this is just how
> some people talk.
>   . . . our message is really simple: We stammer, it's
> how we talk. We need people to simply accept this
> and move away from ideas about how we can or how
> we should change. In this day and age, stammering
> shouldn't be viewed negatively and met with
> suggestions to 'fix it'. It should be embraced and
> acknowledged as simply the way someone speaks."
>   (Stamma website, Oct 2020, accessed April 2021)

As part of this campaign, posters were placed in prominent
places around the United Kingdom and postcards were
produced correcting unhelpful and inappropriate ways of
talking about stammering. Two examples were:

> *Emily Blunt* credits a
> school teacher for
> helping her to ~~overcome~~
> control the **stammer**
> through acting . . .

The way we talk about stammering is wrong so we
worked with Wikipedia to make it right.

> *Joe Biden* has
> ~~had problems with~~

~~stuttering throughout~~
~~all his life~~ a stutter.

The way we talk about stammering is wrong so we worked with Wikipedia to make it right.

This successful campaign illustrates the language used to pathologise stammering but then how simply it can be challenged and changed. This message is one that can be used widely but also applies to everyone in conversation with others.

(Note: In this book, the use of 'person who stammers' [PWS] has been intentionally chosen to reflect the individuality of each person who has a stammer and to put the person before the stammer. It was not intended as a concise way of grouping together those with a particular way of speaking. However, I accept that this may not be the term preferred by some who stammer. Indeed, those affiliated with 'stammering pride' often wish to be referred to as stammerers as a way of aligning themselves directly with the stammering community. It is recommended that those who work alongside individuals with stammering speech ask how they prefer to be addressed when referring to them in writing or speaking.)

i. Disclosure: 'It's OK to stammer'. In previous sections of this book, being open about stammering, stammering openly and talking about it with others were all features of common interventions across a number of approaches (see **Section E, Point 48**). Their inclusion in this section comes from a different place. The purpose of disclosing stammering to others in a 'stammer more proudly' context is to own stammering, proclaim the right to stammer and encourage the rest of the world to embrace it as one of several diverse ways of speaking. While there are benefits to self-disclosure for the PWS, the objective here is to change other people's view of what it is and facilitate *their* desensitisation process, helping them to accept it as simply a different way of talking.

There has been some research on ways in which a PWS could disclose their stammer to others. It is important to separate out the research which is part of the 'speak more fluently' and 'stammer more easily' approaches. For example, Breitenfeldt and Lorenz (1999), in the manual for their Successful Stuttering Management program, outline three ways a PWS may disclose his stammer to a conversational partner:

a. make a direct statement saying he has a stammer at the beginning of the conversation or immediately after a stammer has occurred

b. after stammering, make a joke about it, which, according to the authors, will put the other person at ease

c. carry out a pseudo- or fake stammer (or voluntary stammer) which will advertise the stammer early in the conversation and desensitise the speaker to his stammer.

It is clear from this example that the disclosure here is used for the purpose of desensitising the speaker to his stammer and not to effect change in his conversational partner's attitude to stammering. However, there are other more recent examples, which looked at the effect of some examples of disclosure on listeners, specifically:

a. when the disclosure is made in a conversation (Healey et al. 2007; Lincoln & Bricker-Katz 2008)

b. the different types of disclosure (Byrd, Croft et al. 2017)

c. whether the disclosure was accompanied by a speech modification technique (Lee & Manning 2010).

These studies have relevance to the 'stammer more proudly' movement in that they increase the understanding of what helps the stammering voice be heard by a conversational partner.

In particular, the research by Byrd, Croft et al. (2017) sheds light on how self-disclosure can effect change in the context of a job interview. In this study, participants viewed a video of an interview scenario in which the candidates who stammered introduced themselves to the interviewer in a variety of ways:

a. including an informative self-disclosure statement: 'Before we get started, I want to let you know that I stutter. You may hear me repeat sounds or phrases, but if there is anything that I say that you do not understand, please don't hesitate to ask me.'

b. including an apologetic statement: 'Before we get started, I should let you know that I stutter, so this might be hard in spots, so bear with me.'

    c. no self-disclosure statement: 'I'm really honored to be here'.

The findings suggested that self-disclosing in an informative manner resulted in more positive listener perceptions. In addition, speakers who use an informative statement were considered more friendly and more confident than those who used an apologetic statement. The results could help a PWS in an interview situation change some of the misperceptions of stammering if he were to use an informative self-disclosure (rather than an apologetic statement) at the beginning of his job interview.

  ii. Collaboration. The 'stammer more proudly' movement seeks to promote a stammering community with individuals who stammer and organisations who work to promote and help children and adults who are dysfluent (e.g. British Stammering Association, International Fluency Association etc.) They are keen to work with researchers and hope to affect the research agenda to:

    a. include partnerships between academics and people who stammer

    b. address questions that are of concern to the stammering community

    c. make the results of studies accessible beyond the confines of academia.

The group also wishes to educate future generations of SLTs about 'stammer more proudly' and have it included in the curriculum of undergraduate degree programmes. Finally, they expect to play a role in campaigning and lobbying and in educating the public in general, challenging the stammering stereotypes and enabling a celebration of stammering and difference.

76. THERAPY AND 'STAMMER MORE PROUDLY'

There is a degree of criticism of SLTs as a whole among some supporters of the 'stammer more proudly' approach. (St Pierre 2015). There are certainly questions about the place of therapy when one has this perspective. If stammering is accepted as part of a neurodiverse pattern of speaking, is there a place for speech and language therapy? If stammering is no longer seen as a disorder or a condition requiring modification, then are SLTs no longer required? Can a 'stammer more proudly' approach sit alongside other approaches, or does it stand alone?

Here are the views of some PWS regarding what role SLTs might play:

> "There are so many myths, personal opinions, untruths and misunderstandings about stammering. A specialist SLT who embraces the social model, who can help the PWS navigate their own journey 'to pride'. Negotiating voluntary stammering, 'coming out', acceptance and so much more can all benefit from good SLT support."

> "It is important that the SLT is clear about the social model. It is not 'well here's the social model, it's so important, but let's work on some fluency strategies as well'. No, it should be straight down the line: acceptance, being open, etc.'"

> "I totally believe in the help of experts to sort out issues we many times cannot handle ourselves. I think stammering should be approached from a holistic perspective, with emotional support from psychological therapy (to cover the root of the emotional triggers) and with the help of language therapy to find the best strategies to communicate effectively. However, it is a very personal journey and what is right for one person might not be right for another."

As the 'stammer pride' movement gains momentum, I too have reflected on the role an SLT might play. Currently stammering remains culturally stigmatised; it is not accepted as part of neurodiversity of speech, and those who stammer continue to struggle to be heard. There is a great deal of work to be done within society; with employers, educators, media and so on to change attitudes and practices and to make stammering less oppressed. SLTs have a role to play with individuals who stammer who wish to embrace this challenge and also can engage in a wider lobbying role.

Sam Simpson is an SLT who works within a 'stammering more proudly' model, and this is how she describes her approach to would-be clients. (This description is taken from the www.redefiningstammering.co.uk website.)

> "I believe in . . . working with you to understand how your stammering is influencing your life choices and how you feel about yourself; increasing your communication choices, opportunities and confidence as well as creating a stammer-friendly environment and working with your family, friends, work colleagues and community as you see relevant. I can also offer opportunities to get involved in a broader dialogue about stammering and therapy through blogs, talks and campaigning, if of interest."
>
> (Simpson) [accessed March 2021]

In this section, the role of an SLT in relation to the objectives of stammer pride will be detailed.

i.   Neurodiversity. In order to help a PWS understand stammering as part of the neurodiversity of speech, therapy involves an exploration of difference. Bond (2021) uses models of disability as a starting point.

     An important part of therapy would be exploring and discussing different models of disability and/or initially what the word disability means to the person.

     This would then lead on to consideration of the specific issues around stammering as a disability, for example, looking at the range of types of talking and the variety of speech which is subsumed under the term 'dysfluency' or 'stammering'. Examples can be drawn from the media (and the lack of dysfluent speakers noted), as well as from the person's environment. A client is then invited to explore how he came to see his stammer and the social values, stigma and prejudices which affected his vision. It is recommended to start by looking at the cultural attitudes to language and speaking in general terms, what is valued and what is invalidated, before moving on to the person's own experience. Discussion of early childhood memories, family members talking or not talking about stammering as it developed, school recollections of bullying and teachers' attitudes to dysfluency in the class, further education experiences, job interviews and employers' views of stammering can all be included. Similarly, a person with an acquired stammer may be invited to reflect on his experiences of being a fluent speaker and the value placed on his ability to be fluent. This can be contrasted with his new situation and how society regards him now his speech is less fluent. (In the later part of therapy, the issues raised by these exercises may be something a person wishes to address as part of an empowerment process.)

Using Sheehan's (1958) iceberg metaphor in the context of work on identification, Campbell (2019b) (www.redefiningstammering.co.uk) has talked about considering not only what is above (overt features of stammering) and below (covert features of stammering) the water line of the iceberg but also what is in the sea. He argues that this enables a PWS to understand the genesis of his negative feelings towards his stammer:

> "The iceberg alone makes no attempt to place these negative feelings into the context of societal oppression of stammering in which they are born. Without this context, the person who stammers is left holding a list of perceived personal failures resulting from their stammering. From a social model perspective, we can shift the focus onto the freezing seas of societal prejudice and discrimination towards stammering that cause the formation of the iceberg, to highlight that the iceberg is not 'the fault' of the person who stammers but rather a natural by-product of societal- and self-oppression."
>
> (Campbell 2019b)

Stammering Iceberg

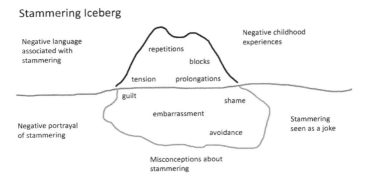

Figure 8.1 The Stammering Iceberg from the Perspective of the Social Model

I think this is a valuable exercise which could be included in the identification exercise using the iceberg (see **Section D, Point 40**) and explored within individual therapy and group settings.

ii. Exploration of the use of language. As discussed previously, part of the genesis of negative attitudes towards stammering comes from the widespread use of terms such as 'overcoming', 'battling with' and 'handicapped by' stammering. It is helpful for a PWS to understand the power that these messages have in relation to society's attitudes and his own experiences around his stammer. A client can be supported in recognising the power language has by reading articles readily available in magazines and newspapers and on the internet about stammering 'cures' and stories of individuals who stammer.

Using the BSA/Stamma editorial guidelines, for example: Don't use negative words.

- People do not 'suffer from' and are not 'afflicted by' stammering. They stammer and live with it.
- A stammer is not a 'weakness' or 'a defect'. It is simply a stammer.
- A stammer is not 'terrible' or 'debilitating'. Moments of stammering might last longer for some.

- People don't 'defeat' or 'overcome' their stammer. They 'manage' it.
  Don't use 'stammering' as a pejorative description. It reinforces the idea that it is bad, and something people shouldn't do. There are other words to describe a failing politician, project or football match.

(accessed July 2021)

Alternatively, using the BSA/Stamma campaign 'Find the Right Words' (see **Point 75**) as an example of challenging and changing the use of unhelpful language around stammering, a PWS may then be invited to talk about the alternative narratives he would like to read and perhaps write one about himself. Burgess (2021), a specialist SLT, said:

"I have found Stamma's Find the Right Words campaign useful and regularly share that to encourage people to notice and call out negative language around stammering which is contributing to the stigma. Also helping people to understand that the reason they might find it difficult to feel positive/proud about their stammer is because of society's negative view of it, which they have internalised, and encouraging them to challenge those long-held beliefs."

(Personal communication 2021)

Owning and valuing stammering. One activity I have used in therapy with both individuals and in a group setting is to have clients identify the advantages and disadvantages of stammering (or the pros and cons). The disadvantages are often easily listed, but proposing that there are advantages to stammering will often raise an eyebrow and in some cases may result in angry outbursts. In the context of stammering pride, the consideration of the benefits of having a stammer is a worthwhile exercise. It is interesting to read several accounts by individuals who have explored this issue themselves, and examples may provide a PWS with a useful starting point for his own reflections.

Rebecca Russell (2020), writing on the Stamma website, said:

> "In a world that tells people to hide their brokenness, I can be the one to prove that you don't have to. I can choose to take joyful pride in my stutter, because I stand out from within a society that prizes perfection."
>
> (accessed April 2021)

In a blog on a stammering website (www.redefiningstammering.co.uk), Aston (2019) talks about reconstruing his stammering and 'luxuriating' in its occurrence. Included in this blog is a painting he produced in response to this desire to stay in his dysfluent moment, which offers an interesting opportunity to present other media for a PWS to use to explore and positively know his stammer.

> "Instead of feeling shame in my speech and in the way my stammer takes temporary control over my body, I would have to seek out my stammer and try to properly experience and picture it. Time after time in the book, and in Stamma's recent successful campaign, it is pointed out that the language we use to describe our stammer is important. I wondered if it would be possible to try to capture a slowed down stammer and almost luxuriate in the moment."
>
> (Aston 2019)

It is an interesting exercise to have a PWS consider 'My stammering self' as a point on a journey to find pride in dysfluency. What does the stammer give to the self that would be missed if it were not there? Alpern (2019) talks of the 'special insight' which stammering gives into language. She says:

> "To the stutterer, spoken words carry a dimension of meaning that's inaccessible to fluent speakers' which can also be ' . . . a place for curiosity, insight, and social connection'."
>
> (p. 19)

In the same text, Constantino (2019) contemplates the 'delight' and 'intimacy' which stammering affords him. He describes the delight in the ability to stammer to transform a mundane, routine greeting of a co-worker into:

> "something unique. The co-worker is forced to connect with me. Perhaps we even have a mean-ingful dialogue! . . . Whether giving a presentation, making a phone call. . . . chances are the other person is not expecting stuttering. This instantly changes the nature of the exchange. It becomes new, curious and singular."
>
> (p. 219)

Regarding intimacy, he writes of the vulnerability which stammering produces. It is this state that Constantino says allows social interactions to be deeper and more intimate:

> "If we allow stuttering to happen, we can invite others to strip and join us. Without all the distraction of fronts and facades we increase our chances of connecting with others and of having worthwhile meaningful conversations."

Mitchell (2016) also talks of his stammer as 'an empathy generator' and sees value in what his stammer has taught and ennobled in him:

> "I'm proud of my knowledge of this tiny, tiny area of the human condition and I wouldn't want to lose it. It makes me more compassionate to other stammerers, of course, but I also believe it gives me a slight connection with other comrades in adversity."

Using these voices and others like them helps a PWS contemplate the added value that a stammer brings to his personal qualities.

iii. Finding a unique way of stammering. There is stammering and then there is what a PWS does to struggle against the stammer and try to prevent it from being heard. In therapy, a PWS can be helped to eliminate or reduce the elements of struggle in his stammer. Bailey (2019) describes her experiences of letting go of the struggle part of her dysfluency and how liberating that process was:

> "when I named what I was doing as struggle the change followed quite naturally. . . . I was helped at the City Lit to become more aware, to become mindful during my struggling and let my dysfluency show."
>
> (p. 31)

Constantino (2021) describes this lack of struggle as the feature of 'spontaneity' which is lacking in the outcome of speech in both the 'speak more fluently' and 'stammer more easily' approaches:

> "I've come to call this quality of speaking spontaneity. It has three characteristics: i) little premeditation, ii) effortless production, and iii) is enjoyable and meaningful.
>
> Spontaneous disfluency is speech that is high in disfluency but low in effort, think of the speech of someone letting themselves stutter easily and openly."

In the same article, Constantino goes on to argue that spontaneity has more impact on a speaker's quality of life than fluency.

For an SLT wishing to help a client reduce struggle and increase spontaneity, there are several fluency modifications which can be used to help. Having gone through an identification process to look at the elements of struggle, the PWS will have his own ideas about areas to focus on which should be given priority. The SLT may offer additional options, for example, all the support mechanisms and prerequisite skills discussed in **Section E, Point 47** are important and of relevance, as are the common interventions in **Points 48–51** (i.e. openness, desensitisation, voluntary stammering and avoidance reduction). In addition, specific techniques to help a PWS reduce backtracking and move forward in their speech (as discussed in **Section G, Points 62 and 65**), such as managing postponements by varying, disrupting run-ins, doubling and so on, can be used, provided the aim is the promotion of struggle-free stammering rather than stammer-less speech.

Assertiveness. The need for a PWS to explore aspects of assertiveness as a prerequisite in therapy was discussed in **Section E, Point 47**. The aim at that early point in therapy was to explore the choices a PWS makes in his communication, including speaking and remaining silent. For example, does the fear of stammering mean that he decides not to speak, or will he assert his right to speak out irrespective of the level of his fluency?

In this stammering pride model of intervention, there is an opportunity to investigate in more detail the rights to speak, be heard and have stammering accepted as part of the person who is talking.

One way of examining the PWS's right to speak is through a Bill of Rights. This is a tool frequently used in assertiveness training but can be adapted here specifically regarding stammering. For example, here is a 'Bill of Rights' which has been changed to increase its relevance to a PWS:

ASSERTIVE BILL OF RIGHTS

(Adapted from: www.winona.edu/resilience/Media/Assertive-Bill-of-Rights-Worksheet.pdf accessed April 2021)

Affirmation: it's OK to stammer

I have the right to speak in MY way, including to:

- express my feelings and opinions appropriately and have them taken seriously by others
- ask for what I want
- disagree with others regardless of their relationship to me
- take the time I need to talk
- say 'no' without feeling guilty
- say 'I don't know'
- be treated with respect and not be taken for granted
- feel all of my emotions (including anger) and express them appropriately
- offer no reasons or excuses for my speech
- be given time and space to ask questions

- set my own priorities, including those regarding my speech
- make mistakes
- change my mind
- make my own decisions and deal with the consequences
- feel good about myself, my speech and my life
- exercise any and all of these rights, without feeling guilty.

Each one of these statements can be discussed with the PWS and its implications considered. For example, point 2 in the bill of rights is 'ask for what I want'. A PWS will often find he is most dysfluent when asking for a particular food item in a takeaway; his favourite sandwich or drink becomes difficult to ask for. Given that the bill of rights establishes his entitlement to ask for what he wants, he can be encouraged to elaborate on what this might mean in practice. Specifically, it could include taking as much time as he needs to, to be respectfully given the time to speak and heard, not to be ridiculed or mocked and to be served in the same way as any other customer. Alternatively, these 16 statements may be viewed as a template and the individual encouraged to develop a more personal bill of rights for his particular set of circumstances. The implications of individualised selection of statements can then be explored in the same way.

Another option would be to use the Disability Rights fact sheet on self-advocacy; Disabilityrightsuk.org (Disability Rights UK Factsheet F77). This may also be used to explore issues with a client.

iv. Disclosure. As discussed in **Point 75**, the purpose of disclosure:

> "is to own stammering, proclaim the right to stammer and encourage the rest of the world to embrace it as one of a number of diverse ways of speaking."

Research has shown that disclosing to others leads to self-empowerment and challenges the stereotypical view of the speaker (Byrd, McGill et al. 2017).

What needs to be unpicked in a therapy context is:
- what to disclose
- when to disclose
- with whom to disclose
- how to disclose.

First, what to disclosure: the PWS is proudly owing his stammer and proclaiming it to his audience. Unlike in the desensitisation examples, the aim is not to put the listener at his ease or reduce the speaker's negative emotions around his dysfluency. Here the stammer is presented for others to hear and accept as this person's individual way of talking.

An interesting study by McGill et al. (2018) explored the wording used by adults who stammered when they were disclosing stammering. The results showed that the majority used statements which were direct and had an educational element such as: 'I sometimes stutter, or block – where I have trouble getting a sound out, so you may hear me do so, or see me look like I'm trying to get a word out.'

In the same study, the authors explored how SLTs worked with clients to formulate self-disclosure statements. The results indicated a brainstorming approach was frequently used, and the outcomes were found to positively empower individuals who stammered.

In therapy, discussions with the PWS can centre around if stammering needs to be introduced or just allowed to exist without explanation. If it is decided to mention it, then a form of wording with some options should be established. For example, 'You may have noticed a break in my talking. It is my stammer.' 'I have a stammer, so I will repeat and get stuck on some words from time to time.' The degree of detail included will vary on the context, but an individual may wish to consider whether to explain what stammering is and any pertinent personal details, such as, 'It is a speech difference with a neurological basis that I have had since I was a child.' Other alternatives would be to tackle misapprehensions and stereotypes head on, with comments such as: 'My stammer is not linked to any anxiety or nervousness' and educate the conversational partner regarding how to react/respond, for example, 'So, give me time to finish and do not complete my sentences for me, as I prefer to speak for myself.'

Apologising for stammering should be avoided, and a therapist can have a conversation with her client about the reasons this is unhelpful. The research article by Healey et al. (2007) could be a topic of discussion for this area, as it illustrates the effect of self-apology on the listener's perception of the speaker.

Some individuals in certain contexts feel it is okay to make light of their stammer, and again it is useful to explore the implications and consequences of humorous comments.

Whatever is decided, it is crucial that the form of words used to disclose stammering be devised by the PWS and not imposed by the therapist. This is the client's disclosure, not a therapist-mediated version.

When to disclose: Several research papers on this topic indicate the power of self-disclosure when it is carried out at the beginning of a conversation and/or interview situation (Byrd, McGill et al. 2017). In addition, consideration should be given to whether the PWS considers the self-disclosure helpful and/or necessary to enhance his own feelings of stammering pride.

With whom to disclose: Self-disclosure appears to have a positive impact when used with people who are unknown to the PWS and who are unaware that he has a stammer. Consequently, an individual can positively impact how others will view him, that is, as more friendly, outgoing, and confident (Byrd, McGill et al. 2017), by using self-disclosure.

How to disclose: Finally, a therapist can help a PWS get the most out of a self-disclosure by working on his non-verbal communication. Ideas to portray a confident, assertive persona can be experimented with, followed by roleplay and discussions of whether to include voluntary stammering/pseudo-stammering should the speaker experience more fluency in the moment of the disclosure.

Empowerment. As a PWS increases in his confidence to 'stammer more proudly', a therapist can suggest and create new opportunities for him to speak about stammering in settings outside those in which he routinely talks. He will have talked to family members, friends and possibly others around his social groups, but there will also be options to talk in his workplace or educational institution and in groups with wider impact, for example, formal speaking groups, such as Toastmasters and talks to community groups.

An SLT will be able to signpost him to possibilities to contribute to stammering open days, International Stammering Awareness day (annually on October 22nd), online blogs, conferences and public awareness campaigns such as those organised by the BSA. Stamma/BSA also invites people of all ages to write narratives and send their contributions to the charity for publication on their website.

From time to time, television and radio stations are interested in airing a story about stammering. SLT departments are often contacted to provide the 'expert' voice on the topic of stammering. While I and colleagues have frequently, albeit reluctantly, appeared in this role, I would now think very hard about the appropriateness of participating as representing the voice of stammering. It seems to me that the stammering community must represent themselves and have their dysfluencies heard widely across a variety of platforms. It can be helpful in promoting empowerment for an SLT to stand back or step out and allow the PWS to take his place in the foreground. This is a view shared by other specialist SLTs:

"I have also thought that the more society hears stammering speech the more it becomes desensitised to listening to differences in fluency, so I've encouraged folks to speak up in as many public situations as possible including the media and educational settings. My vision would be to grow this not only in high profile work settings such as the defense stammering network and all the work of the Employers Stammering Network etc. – all signposted by the BSA, but also in factories and other tough workplaces."

(Hansley 2021)

SLTs and others wishing to support a PWS may struggle to know just what to do to help. The National Stuttering Association (NSA) has produced a useful poster entitled 'What does it mean to be an ally to people who stutter?' https://westutter.org/wp-content/uploads/2016/11/Allies. pdf [accessed July 14th, 2021]. It encompasses five sections of advice:

- demonstrating interest and asking open-ended questions about stammering
- respecting that each PWS has unique preferences and perspectives on stammering
- an example of how to model responding to stammering.

v. Psychological strengthening: There are other forms of help and support an SLT can provide to a PWS seeking to develop a 'stammer more proudly' way of living his life. These centre around ways of nurturing, thickening and giving new energy to various psychological processes.

These ideas will be included in the next section, **Section I, Psychological Approaches**.

Finally, this is a relatively new approach and specialist SLTs are working out the part they might play. An interesting article by Bond (2019), 'Speech and Language Therapy and the Social Model: Out at Sea and Lost?', describes her struggles and developing confidence when embracing this in her work and may be an encouragement to others in a similar position.

REFERENCES

Alpern, E. (2019). Why stutter more? In P. Campbell, C. Constantino & S. Simpson (eds.), *Stammering: Pride & Prejudice*. Guilford: J & R Press.

Aston, P. (2019). A sea change. www.redefiningstammering. co.uk [Accessed April 2021].

Bailey, K. (2019). Scary canary: Difference, vulnerability and letting go of struggle. In P. Campbell, C. Constantino & S. Simpson (eds.), *Stammering: Pride & Prejudice*. Guilford: J & R Press.

Bond, K. (2019). Speech and language therapy and the social model: Out at sea and lost? www.redefiningstammering. co.uk [Accessed April 2021].

Bond, K. (2021). *Personal Communication*.

Breitenfeldt, D.H. & Lorenz, D.R. (1999). *Successful Stuttering Management Program (SSMP): For Adolescent and Adult Stutterers*, 2nd edition. Cheney, WA: Eastern Washington University Press.

British Stammering Association. Editorial guidelines. https:// stamma.org/sites/default/files/2021-03/Editorial%20 guidelines%20for%20talking%20about%20 stammering.pdf [Accessed July 2021].

Burgess, S. (2021). *Personal Communication*.

Byrd, C.T., Croft, R., Gkalitsiou, Z. & Hampton, E. (2017). Clinical utility of self-disclosure for adults who stutter: Apologetic versus informative statements. *Journal of Fluency Disorders*, 54, 1–13.

Byrd, C.T., McGill, M., Gkalitsiou, Z. & Cappellini, C. (2017). The effects of self-disclosure on male and female perceptions of individuals who stutter. *American Journal of Speech-Language Pathology*, 26, 1, 69–80.

Campbell, P. (2018). Fresh eyes on a well worn path: Re-visiting stammering therapy with the social model and stammering pride. Blog on RedefiningStammering.co.uk [Accessed March 2021].

Campbell, P. (2019a). The origins of stammering pride & prejudice. *Stamma website (British Stammering Association) website* [Accessed 2021].

Campbell, P. (2019b). Re-imagining adult stammering therapy. www.redefiningstammering.co.uk [Accessed April 2021].

Claypole, J. (2021). *Words Fail Us: In Defence of Disfluency*. London: Profile Books Ltd.

Cole, P. (2020). We need to adjust the language and reactions to stammering. *Stamma website. British Stammering Association* [Accessed April 2021].

Constantino, C. (2019). Stuttering naked. In P. Campbell, C. Constantino & S. Simpson (eds.), *Stammering: Pride & Prejudice*. Guilford: J & R Press.

Constantino, C. (2021). Spontaneous stuttering. Blog on www.redefiningstammering.co.uk [Accessed March 2021].

Hansley, E.C. (2021). *Personal Communication*.

Healey, E.C., Gabel, R.M., Daniels, D.E. & Kawai, N. (2007). The effects of self-disclosure and non self-disclosure of stuttering on listeners' perceptions of a person who stutters. *Journal of Fluency Disorders*, 32, 51–69.

Hunt, P. (1966). *Stigma: The Experience of Disability*. London: Geoffrey Chapman.

Johnson, J.K. (2008). The visualization of the twisted tongue: Portrays of stuttering in film, television and comic books. *Journal of Popular Culture*, 45, 245–261.

Lee, K. & Manning, W. (2010). Listener responses according to stuttering self-acknowledgment and modification. *Journal of Fluency Disorders*, 35, 110–122.

Lincoln, M. & Bricker-Katz, G. (2008). Self-disclosure of stuttering at the beginning of interactions may improve listeners' perceptions of people who stutter. *Evidence Based Communication Assessment and Intervention*, 2, 87–89.

McGill, M., Siegel, J., Nguyen, D. & Rodriguez, S. (2018). Self-report of self-disclosure statements for stuttering. *Journal of Fluency Disorders*, 58, 22–34.

Mitchell, D. (2016). *Thirteen Ways of Looking at a Stammer*. Germany: Stotteren & Selbsthilfe Landesverband Ost e. V.

Oliver, M. (1990). *The Politics of Disablement*. London: Macmillan Publishers Ltd.

Pierre, J. (2019). An introduction to stuttering and disability theory: Misfits in meaning. In P. Cambell, C. Constantino & S. Simpson (eds.), *Stammering Pride & Prejudice*. Guilford: J & R Press.

Russell, R. (2020). Am I really proud to stammer? *Stamma Website British Stammering Association* [Accessed April 2021].

Sheehan, J.G. (1958). Conflict theory and avoidance reduction therapy. In J. Eisenson & O. Bloodstein (eds.), *Stuttering: A Symposium*. New York: Harper.

Simpson, S., Cambell, P. & Constantino, C. (2021). *Stammering: Difference not Defect*. Oxford: Oxford Dysfluency Conference Presentation.

Stewart, T. (1995). Efficacy of speech and language therapy for fluency disorders: Adults who stammer. *International Journal of Language and Communication*, 30, S1, 478–483.

St Pierre, J. (2015). Dis-counting speech: Why are we still measuring stuttering? www.didistutter.org [Accessed 2 August 2021].

Section I

PSYCHOLOGICAL APPROACHES

77. THE ROLE PSYCHOLOGICAL APPROACHES PLAY IN THE MANAGEMENT OF STAMMERING

Stammering should not be regarded as a psychological disorder. (The current evidence for a genetic and/or neurological cause for stammering is substantial.) Rather, stammering has an effect on the person which often results in the development of psychological issues in adolescence and adulthood. It is these secondary features which can be helped by a number of psychological approaches which will be discussed in this section.

78. WHAT KIND OF PSYCHOLOGICAL ISSUES CAN DEVELOP IN AN ADOLESCENT AND ADULT WHO STAMMERS?

The effect of stammering on emotional and mental health has been documented extensively. Several articles have reviewed this data with a focus on anxiety (Bloodstein & Bernstein Ratner 2008; Craig & Tran 2006; Menzies et al. 1999).

In addition, there are a number of other studies which have investigated the impact of stammering on quality of life (QOL) measures. Klompas and Ross (2004) found a negative influence on emotional stability and self-esteem. Both Klompas and Ross and Craig et al. (2009) found that adults who stammered, when compared to adults who did not stammer, had lower QOL scores on measures of:

- vitality, resulting in increased risks of being fatigued (a state associated with feelings of distress and poor mood)

 DOI: 10.4324/9781003177890-10

- social functioning, suggesting a negative impact on social interaction capacity
- emotional role functioning
- mental health.

With regard to the frequency of stammering, Andrade et al. (2008) reported in their study that both mild and severe stammering had negative effects on QOL, while Koedoot et al. (2011) reported moderate to severe stammering had negative effects on overall QOL.

Other studies have identified the psychological impact of living with a stammer. Notably, Corcoran and Stewart (1998), in an interesting qualitative study of the stories of adults who stammered, investigated the experiences of 14 adults. They discovered that suffering was the primary theme of the narratives, which resulted in feelings of helplessness, shame, fear and avoidance. These findings were echoed in a study carried out by Crichton-Smith (2002). She found the key elements of the experience of stammering to be suffering, helplessness, shame and stigma, but these features occurred at different stages and to varying degrees in a person's life.

79. WHAT TO DO?

From as far back as the 1950s, writers have been discussing psychological approaches to the issues associated with stammering (Williams 1957). Later, Van Riper's (1973) approaches to treatment of stammering reflected his awareness and concern for client's level of anxiety, fear, frustration and shame.

While the evidence for the occurrence of psychological issues alongside the overt features of stammering appears undeniable, some SLTs appear to be disinclined to address them with a PWS, perhaps feeling ill equipped or believing such interventions to be the responsibility of other professionals.

"many clinicians seem to be reluctant to address these more covert aspects or express a low comfort level in dealing with attitudes related to the complex problem of stuttering. This reluctance or discomfort may be due in part to an overall lack of confidence in working with people who stutter. . . . Moreover, many clinicians have little or no formal training in counseling and, hence, feel ill prepared to deal with attitudinal issues"

(Watson 1995, p. 144)

However, there are approaches that can be carried out by an inexperienced SLT working with adults who stammer which are effective and should be an important part of the holistic management of dysfluency. In Blood's The POWER game (1995) designed for use with adolescents and adults, he deals with a number of areas designed to develop resilience. These include: problem-solving, negotiating, self-esteem, control, social support and responsibility. Several writers emphasise the need for work on attitudes and cognitions alongside other speech modification approaches (Cooper & Cooper 1995; Daly et al. 1995). Everard (2019) wrote:

"We believe that stammering results from a complex interaction of attitudes, thoughts, feelings and behaviours, with avoidance of stammering playing a key role in maintaining stammering. It is therefore essential in therapy to address emotional, attitudinal and avoidance aspects of stammering as well as the speech itself."

(p. 16)

A number of particular psychological interventions require specific training, which can be accessed by the relevant training institution and will prove a vital part of a therapist's array of resources. The remainder of this section will outline some types of interventions which should be considered.

80. MINDFULNESS

There are some misunderstandings about what mindfulness entails. To be clear, mindfulness is not another form of relaxation and does not involve emptying the mind of thoughts. Mindfulness practice is, however, about:

> 🏮 I wish I had known that mindfulness can work. It is not pseudoscience.
> Jon-Øivind Finbråten (Personal Communication 2021)

> "paying attention in a particular way: on purpose, in the present moment and nonjudgmentally."
>
> (Kabat-Zinn 1994, p. 4)

and:

> "a radical non-doing, inviting a counter-intuitive inward stance of acceptance and opening rather than fixing or problem solving."
>
> (Kabat-Zinn 2005)

Boyle (2011), drawing from Baer et al. (2004), stated:

> "Mindfulness is a multifaceted construct that includes observation of inner and outer experiences (e.g. noticing when one's mood begins to change), acting with awareness (e.g. noticing the mind wandering and becoming distracted when doing an activity), and acceptance of internal and external phenomena (e.g. not being judgmental of oneself for feeling negative emotions)."
>
> (p. 123)

Boyle goes on to describe how mindfulness can be developed through the practice of meditation and informal practice of:

• 'focused attention' on, for example, breathing
• 'open monitoring', which involves being aware of, for example, thoughts, feelings and bodily sensations.

Mindfulness, according to Cheasman (2021), is a trainable skill, and she has described an eight-week mindfulness-based cognitive therapy programme for adults who stammer (2013). She described the aims of mindfulness-based approaches as:

- the development of insight and awareness
- the increase in the possibility of choice through responding mindfully rather than reacting automatically
- the cultivation of acceptance
- the increase in kindness and compassion towards self
- the increase in the possibility of experiencing calm.

These aims are achieved through:

- an increase in awareness, leading to making choices to respond rather than reacting on autopilot
- change coming about through letting be rather than trying to fix
- a positive approaching and opening up to difficult experiences which can reduce the reactive pattern of tensing, which triggers negative cycles of thoughts, feelings and behaviours
- a disengaging from rumination and habituated negative thinking patterns.

When applied to stammering, several writers have detailed how mindfulness can help. The psychosocial and sensory-motor benefits encompass exposure to internal and external experiences which may be routinely avoided, 'improved emotional regulation', enhanced attention to the present moment, acceptance of stammering and better understanding of the power of thought (Boyle 2011). Reduction of fear and anxiety and an increase in positive attitudes to speaking, locus of control and problem-focused coping behaviours have been reported by Fairburn et al. (2009). Drawing on his personal, regular mindfulness practice, Brocklehurst [accessed May 2021] listed a number of ways in which he has benefitted, including identification of his stammering behaviours and listener reactions to stammering, reduction in unhelpful value judgements he has made about his speaking, reduction of secondary symptoms (such as avoidance and 'escape' behaviours) and development of self-esteem.

When using mindfulness with a PWS, a therapist may consider using a whole programme, such as described by Cheasman (2013). Alternatively, she can use mindfulness activities to ground an individual at the beginning of a session, such as feet on floor, body on chair (Cheasman 2021), or to enable emotional regulation when something powerful has been evoked during a session and/or at the end of a session to help the person transition from therapy into the remainder of his day.

There are a number of scripted mindfulness practices available for an SLT new to this work on the following websites: www.mindfulhealth.co.uk, www.bangor.ac.uk and www.umassmed.edu/cfm.

In addition, the following are activities recommended when working with an adult who stammers:

i.   focused attention. The raisin exercise is an experiential introduction to mindfulness. A full description and script can be found in Cheasman (2021).
ii. body scan. In this practice, the person focuses his attention on parts of the body in turn. The attention is held for a few moments and any sensations explored before moving on to the next area. A full description can be found in Cheasman (2021).

> "The body scan has applications for PWS because it may increase awareness of tension associated with thoughts and feelings related to speaking and stuttering. Increased awareness of bodily sensations may improve self-monitoring of the muscles used in speech and likely facilitate easier speech production."
> (Boyle 2011, p. 126)

iii. Breathing meditations. Segal et al. (2002) recommended the use of a short grounding exercise called 'the three-step breathing space' and an elaboration called 'the responding breathing space'. This practice enables a person to reconnect with the present through noticing his thoughts, feelings and body sensations. Full descriptions of both practices with links to audio files can be found in Cheasman (2021).

iv. Changing a person's relationship to his thoughts. Thoughts can exert a great deal of power over a person. Learning to change the relationship he has with his thoughts and no longer see them as 'truths' enables a PWS to take more control. Segal et al. (2002) recommend:
- watching thoughts come and go without following them
- viewing thoughts as a series of mental events rather than facts to be acted upon
- writing thoughts down so distance is found between the thought and any emotion
- looking at the origin of the thought and its relevance to the current situation.

v. When a PWS is in the action phase of therapy, Segal et al. (2002) also suggest a mindful approach in which the individual takes a breathing space. This pause in his action enables him to increase his awareness required for decision making. He then considers the best course of action for the situation.

vi. Finally, the same writers, Segal et al. (2002), have a mindful approach to the time when the individual finds it difficult to maintain the gains he has made. This is a stage which the client prepares for (see **Section J**). Included in the plan are the identification of factors associated with setbacks, increasing the person's ability to identify their emergence and engaging others in this early identification. A three-step plan for managing these occurrences is outlined:
- take a three-minute breathing space
- make a choice based on past experience to ground the self
- take some action or perform an activity which facilitates empowerment and mastery in the situation.

81. ACCEPTANCE AND COMMITMENT THERAPY

i. Defining acceptance. What does acceptance mean in this context? The notion of acceptance within acceptance and commitment therapy (ACT) is based on Harris (2009):

"acceptance means allowing our thoughts and feelings to be as they are, regardless of whether they are pleasant or painful, opening up and making room for them, dropping the struggle with them and letting them come and go and do as they naturally do."

(p. 134)

In relation to stammering, the key here is the PWS being with his difficulty and wholly embracing it rather than waging a war against it with tension, avoidance and struggle behaviours. Plexico et al. (2009) stated that:

"Acceptance involves acknowledging to the self and others that a problem exists, that the problem does not define the speaker's identity, and the individual is capable of being an active agent in the change process."

(p. 121)

The aims of ACT. With mindfulness at its core, ACT has two main aims:
• to help create a full, rich and meaningful life whilst accepting the pain that inevitably comes with it
• to teach mindfulness skills that allow more effective management of painful thoughts and feelings, thereby reducing their impact.

Using ACT with PWS: ACT has been used with a wide range of clients, but, in a review of ACT programmes, Beilby and Byrnes (2012) showed its relevance for stammering management. Other studies have documented its usefulness for adults who stammer (Beilby & Byrnes 2010a, 2010b; Byrnes et al. 2010).

Plexico et al. (2005) noticed that acceptance was a key factor in the process of change in adults who stammered. In a further study exploring the nature of coping strategies of persons who stammered, Plexico et al. (2009) found acceptance an important factor and an impetus for:

"greater self understanding, increased cognitive and affective comfort, more comfortable relationships with others, and less of a need for self-concealment provided by coping patterns characterized by avoidance and escape."

(p. 121)

Furthermore, Yaruss (2012) affirmed acceptance as an active process which should be a primary therapy goal:

"Speakers who have achieved greater acceptance of stuttering not only find it easier to communicate, but also easier to live the life they want to live."

(p. 187)

Cheasman et al. (2015) place acceptance at the heart of their therapeutic relationship with clients, especially the non-judgmental, non-stereotyping and careful use of language when referring to stammering and the PWS.

Moreover, Everard and Cheasman (2021) regard a number of established therapy practices as having acceptance at their core, specifically identification, desensitisation, avoidance reduction and aspects of block modification:

"The integration of ACT into adult stammering therapy supports work on increased awareness of both overt and covert elements of stammering, avoidance-reduction, becoming more open to the experience of stammering, speech change, and motivation to keep going in challenging situations."

(p. 164)

ii. Talking about ACT with PWS: Recognising the difficulty with the term, Cheasman et al. (2015) recommend a number of alternative terms when discussing this with a client. For example, 'allowing things to be here', 'letting be', 'making space for' and 'opening up to'. In addition, the concepts of 'friendly curiosity' and 'willingness' are proposed, as they indicate an alternative to resistance and struggle.

iii. Psychological flexibility. The development of psychological flexibility is fundamental to ACT. This is accomplished through the application of six core processes:
   • self-concept, i.e. how the person views and defines themselves

- defusion, i.e. behavioural flexibility
- acceptance, i.e. embracing emotional and cognitive events without attempting to change them
- mindfulness, i.e. focusing on the present moment rather than past experiences
- values, i.e. clarifying the areas of life which hold the most meaning
- committed action, i.e. establishing goals and quality of life priorities for the future.

(Beilby & Byrnes 2012)

These core processes have been subsumed into three pillars by Flaxman et al. (2019). A therapist can facilitate an individual to move through these processes organically, as he needs, rather than in a linear way.

a. the Noticing Pillar. Noticing can be developed through mindfulness. In ACT, mindfulness generally has three basis tenets: notice, let go of the thought, let feelings be. (For further discussion of mindfulness, see the previous **Point 80** in this section.)

b. the Open Pillar. In the Open Pillar, a person works on developing new and different reactions to his problematic thoughts and feelings. According to Flaxman et al. (2019), this can be done in three ways: becoming aware of unhelpful thoughts, taking thoughts less seriously and creating space between oneself and thoughts. Defusion and acceptance are the key components of the open pillar (Cheasman 2021).

c. the Active Pillar. In the Active Pillar, the PWS will develop an understanding of his values: those which are personal to him and can be expressed in his everyday life. He will be enabled to take these values forward into committed action and manage any procrastination, anxiety and the expectations of others which may be holding him back.

iv. An ACT programme for a PWS has been devised and reported on by Beilby et al. (2012) The programme consisted of eight two-hour sessions delivered in a group therapy setting. All six core processes described previously were included. The sessions were organised as follows:

Session 1: familiarised the client with ACT and identified therapeutic goals linked to the client's values

Session 2: increased the client's awareness of emotional control as well as the consequences of control efforts. This session included an introduction to the concepts of willingness and acceptance as alternatives to experiential avoidance

Session 3: worked on identification of private events to target for defusion and acceptance

Session 4: further extended defusion work and expanded the mindfulness skills into daily life

Session 5: addressed the completion of defusion, extended the mindfulness training and clarified the client's personal set of values

Session 6: instigated committed action and management of client-identified barriers to such action

Session 7: promoted continuation of value-directed activities; that is, participants were asked to identify areas of their life which were most meaningful and the personal resources which were focused on coping with and avoiding negative life experiences and to refocus on achieving defined personal values

Session 8: processed the reactions of the client to the conclusion of the treatment program, reviewed the ACT strategies and techniques and set goals to promote post-treatment maintenance of therapeutic gains.

82. PERSONAL CONSTRUCT PSYCHOLOGY AND THERAPY

i. Theoretical basis. Based on the writings of George Kelly, personal construct psychology (PCP) has been applied to stammering since the 1970s and 80s: Fransella (1972), Evesham and Fransella (1985), Evesham and Huddleston (1983) and Hayhow and Levy (1989). PCP can help to explain and manage some of the barriers to change that a PWS may encounter in therapy, such as adjusting to a new speaker role.

The theory is based on Kelly's (1955) idea of the person as a scientist: the individual who is constantly formulating hypotheses about how the future will be and seeking evidence to test out his predictions. He develops and uses a bipolar set of personal constructs which are organised into a hierarchical system and help him in his predictions.

"As is clear from Kelly's description of construct systems, people use these systems to organize their world in order to be better able to understand it and to predict and control the course of future events. As new experience creates the need to review certain constructs so as to provide a better fit for the system, existing constructs may be altered."

(DiLollo et al. 2002, p. 23)

These constructs may be tight, that is, less open to change, or loose and able to be altered. Either of these extremes has its own issues, as a tight system of constructs is difficult to change, where as a looser arrangement makes it hard for the person to make any workable predictions.

ii. Applying PCP to stammering. In one of the first studies to apply PCP to stammering, Fransella (1972) hypothesised that a PWS continues to stammer because in this way he can anticipate the greatest number of events and consequently is more able to construe or understand his life:

"Fransella's argument is that people who stutter will be able to predict the variety of ways in which a particular person will react to their speaking, the ways that they will react to their own speech, and the ways in which they will react to the listener's reactions to their speaking. On the other hand, persons who stutter know little about how events will proceed if they speak fluently; they are inexperienced in interpreting normal reactions to fluent speech."

(DiLollo et al. 2002, p. 24)

Other studies using PCP (Dalton 1983, 1994; Williams 1995) have explored how a PWS does not give the same weight to his experience of fluent speech as he does to stammering. In my clinical work, I recall a client who was able to control his speech in clinic very effectively but reverted to a less fluent speaking mode in other settings. In a spirit of curiosity, I asked him about this, and in his reply he described how his more fluent voice 'didn't feel like me'. (This was a significant conversation for me, and I realised the need to understand where stammering and changes in speech fitted into a person's understanding of himself. I went on to learn about and use PCT in my work with individuals who stammered.) Dalton noted the difference in how individuals who stammered described their stammering experience but struggled to put into words their awareness of feelings of control. In a later study, she observed that having a PWS describe himself apart from his stammer gave the opportunity for him to begin to elaborate a fuller picture of himself.

iii. PCT and stammering therapy. The use of PCT by a trained SLT can enable a number of possibilities:

- to understand the client's psychological view of the world. This, as Williams (1995) wrote, has allowed therapists:

"to understand, almost, what it is like to stutter and to appreciate the implications of change for clients."

(p. 111)

- to explore the client's view of his stammer and how and why it gives meaning to him
- to provide new alternatives or ways of construing for the PWS to explore
- to provide a creative cycle of hypothesis formulation and testing, experimentation, re-evaluation and reconstruing on the basis of the experimenting.

(This replaces the old formulae of practice-failure-recrimination-more practice [Hayhow & Levy 1989], which is a cycle recognised by many adults who stammer who have previous experiences of therapy.)

"the process of personal construct counselling is the process of understanding the client's construing of the world as seen through the eyes of personal construct theory and thereby, being in a position to facilitate the client's reconstruing of life and experience."

(Fransella & Dalton 1990, p. 6)

Stewart and Brosh (1997) describe the interaction with a client using PCT and art therapy. The individual was able to move from an initial place of isolation and desperation (see Image 1) through to the consideration of possibilities and weighing up of choices (see Image 2) to a final point of social engagement, albeit with a sense of vulnerability (see Image 3).

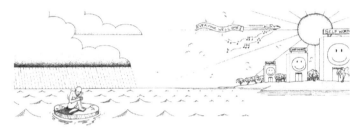

Image 1 Beginning Therapy, Client M.

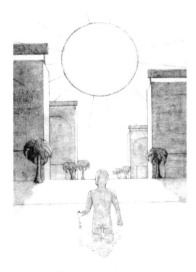

Image 2 Mid-Point in Therapy, Client M.

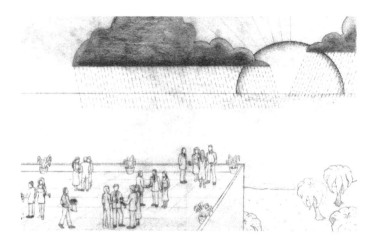

Image 3 At the End of Therapy, Client M.

iv. Benefits of using PCT with PWS.
  a. Clarity. PCT allows the clinician and client to see stammering in the context of his understanding of himself and his world. Thus, therapy has greater relevance and personal meaning for him. (See Stewart and Birdsall [2001] for a client's description of personal change through PCT.)
  b. The use of PCT with a PWS is an holistic way of approaching the issues of stammering. PCT not only addresses thoughts and feelings regarding speaking but also asks the person to experiment with his behaviours in order to bring about change. Fransella and Dalton (1990) discuss the process of change in a PCP model:

> "this is not just a matter of changing a person's way of thinking about things . . . it is in action, in the person's experiments with ways of behaving differently that new constructions of events are tried and tested."
>
> (p. 105)

  c. PCT can be effectively used with other speech modifications. Fransella (1972) felt that a PCP approach was most beneficial after a client had managed to achieve a degree of control over his speech. This control would then allow him to experiment with alternative actions in social and speaking situations. Williams (1995) also stressed the effective links between behavioural experimentation and reconstruction. However, PCT can also be used in isolation to bring about change without additional speech modification, such as 'speak more fluently' or 'stammer more easily' approaches. A person can reconstrue how he feels about himself and his speech in such a way as to mitigate against the need for additional speech change. As such, it is a psychological process that sits well alone and alongside the 'stammer more proudly' movement.

d.   Significant change. PCT can enable significant and long-term change. In PCP, Kelly (1955) discusses a number of cycles of construing. One, the 'creativity cycle', is concerned with a process of construing that moves backward and forward from loose to tight construing until a person feels something has been 'created' with which he can experiment.

> "Loosened construction . . . sets the stage for creative thinking. . . . The loosening releases facts, long taken as self-evident, from their conceptual moorings. Once so freed, they may be seen in new aspects hitherto unsuspected, and the creative cycle may get underway."
> (Kelly 1955, p. 1031)

Experience shows that a PWS who has been involved in a process of experimentation and altering construing can continue to work on risk taking, avoidance reduction and confrontation of fears and anxieties over time. Stewart (1996) explored the relationship between long term maintenance of therapy gains and the construing process. Clients who had continued with a looser, more open construct system for longer during group therapy were found to have better maintenance of outcomes. She recommended that clinicians should use more loosening techniques for longer to ensure better maintenance of therapy benefits.

83. COGNITIVE BEHAVIOURAL THERAPY

i. Background. Cognitive therapy was developed by Beck as a short-term therapy for depression in adults and has been used subsequently for a range of emotional issues. It shares some similarities with PCP, which Beck saw as a precursor to CBT. The basic premise of CBT is that emotional reactions and behaviour are influenced by cognitions. Beck proposed that each person was engaged in trying to make sense of his world by organising and interpreting information. Generally, this is useful to him and helps him to predict events. However, on occasion, he can have unhelpful biases at the heart of his interpretation process and, as a result, develops negative or troublesome thought patterns. These thoughts, opinions and interpretations about himself will influence his emotional state and can give rise to difficulties.

ii. The vicious circle. Beck hypothesised that there were connections between thoughts, feelings and physiological and behavioural responses. For example, if I experience anxiety over an imminent event, it will trigger some physiological responses such as increased heart and breathing rate and sweating. In turn, my cognitions may flit quickly from one thought to another or become fixed on a particular physiological experience, such as the increased heart rate. I can develop feelings of panic as my concerns over my heart rate become overwhelming. There may be feelings of fight or flight. If the latter alternative is chosen, a person can develop avoidance around the trigger situation or event. There is a short-term gain as the individual circumvents the difficulty, but ultimately it prevents him from testing out his predictions and discovering that the event was not as problematic as he thought and he could have got through it adequately. When a person repeatedly avoids, his fear and anxiety will increase, and he is likely to lose confidence while developing emotions such as shame and guilt.

iii. What does CBT do? The aim of CBT is to enable a person to, first, identify his unhelpful thought patterns and then to test the truth of these cognitions. Once it is established that the thoughts are obstructive in some way, then the person goes on to develop and test new, more useful lines of thinking. Turnbull and Stewart (2017) summarise the overall approach:

> "It is structured, goal-orientated and collaborative with its emphasis on changing unhelpful thoughts and replacing them with more helpful ones. It is more concerned with how problems are maintained than on how they are caused and, wherever possible, the focus of therapy is in the present rather than the past."
>
> (p. 9)

iv. Why use CBT with a PWS? The ability to manage stammering appears to be related in part to changes in a person's cognition. In a phenomenological study, Plexico et al. (2005) reported that adults who were successfully managing their stuttering found that:

> I would have like to understand the importance of CBT in stuttering treatment. When I understood the fundamentals and the basis of CBT it was easy to apply them to stuttering treatment.
> Monica Rocha (Personal Communication 2021)

> "Transitioning from a life dominated by the theme of stuttering to one in which stuttering was successfully managed required both cognitive and behavioural change."
>
> (p. 14)

The core component of CBT for people who stutter is challenging unhelpful beliefs. For a PWS, these beliefs may be related to:

- anxiety about speaking, e.g. 'I'm going to run out of air/ not be able to breathe.' 'I'll block and not be able to get out of it.'
- possible negative evaluations by others, e.g. 'If I stammer, they will think I'm stupid.' 'People will laugh.'

These unhelpful thoughts will then give rise to physiological responses such as tension and shortness of breath, anxiety reactions, possible panic, avoidance and emotions such as shame and self-depreciation. Iverach et al. (2017) found that maintenance of social anxiety in stammering could be influenced by a host of interrelated factors, including fear of negative evaluation, negative social-evaluative cognitions, attentional biases, self-focused attention, safety behaviours and anticipatory and post-event processing. Craig and Tran (2006) called specifically for the use of cognitive behavioural therapy for all adults who stammered.

v. Evidence for using CBT for stammering issues. Early studies explored the use of CBT to change the negative attitudes of some adults who stammered and develop more optimistic perspectives (Andrews & Craig 1982; Craig & Andrews 1985; Howie et al. 1981; Maxwell 1982). Blood (1995) evaluated the efficacy of a program which combined a commercially available computer-assisted biofeedback program for the reduction of stuttering and a cognitive-based relapse management program for counselling and attitude change. Results show that four young adults reduced their stammering and increased their positive feelings and attitudes. Gains were maintained at a 12-month follow-up. In their report of the ISTAR Comprehensive Stuttering Program, Langevin et al. (2006) describe the use of a number of CBT components in a report of the ISTAR programme, aimed at improving social skills, developing positive attitudes towards communication, reducing avoidance, managing fear and anxiety and dealing with negative listener reactions. Menzies and colleagues (2008) examined the effects on anxiety and stuttering through a CBT package for social anxiety.

vi. How to use CBT with a PWS. First, a clinician should always work within her set of competencies. When considering using CBT, she will have had the necessary training to equip her with the knowledge and skills to employ this approach appropriately. A series of sessions of CBT can be part of an ongoing management programme or may be used in isolation. As stated previously, the aim of such sessions is to identify and modify the negative thoughts and biases the person has in relation to his stammering.

The first step is for the client and therapist to develop an understanding of the problem and the patterns of unhelpful thoughts which the person is experiencing. This may be done by enabling the individual to explore the links between his thoughts, feelings, physiological reactions and behavioural responses. The notion of the vicious circle can help this process. A worked example can be found in Turnbull and Stewart (2017). In addition, the PWS will be asked to evaluate which of his usual ways of coping are helpful and which are less beneficial. Turnbull and Stewart (2017) suggest using Socratic questioning, 'open, collaborative, non-confrontational and. . . . curious questions', as a method of facilitating this process. The PWS may be introduced to unhelpful patterns (such as all-or-nothing thinking, catastrophising, mental filters, mind reading, overgeneralisation, post-mortem thinking, worst-case scenario) in order that he can better identify these in his own thinking.

Second, a client is asked to adopt a critical attitude to his thoughts and to question their validity by identifying, noting and then posing a number of questions, such as:

- what evidence do I have that the thought is correct?
- what evidence do I have that the thought is wrong?
- what would I tell a friend, if they had the same thought, that would help them?
- what would a very understanding and supportive friend say to help me eliminate this thought?
- do I think I am worrying unnecessarily about something that I have no control over?
- how does the thought make me feel – good or bad?
- are there benefits to me giving up thinking this thought? If so, what are they?
- what is the worst outcome that could occur if this thought were true?
- is there an alternative thought I could have that would be more helpful?

Finally, the PWS uses behavioural experiments to establish more helpful thoughts which have been identified as more useful based on his evidence. Bennet-Levy et al. (2004) divide these experiments into two categories:

- active: in which once the unhelpful thought has been identified, the PWS deliberately acts or thinks in a different manner in a problem situation
- observational: often used when performing an action creates too much anxiety or when further evidence is needed.

A checklist, 'Unhelpful Thoughts and Beliefs about Stuttering' (St Clare et al. 2009) (see **Appendix 2**), has formed the basis for CBT worksheets. (Menzies et al. 2009) Full details of the worksheets are included in **Appendix 2**. Questions 1 and 2 on the worksheet focus on the evidence for the negative thought. Question 5 relates to the issues that a PWS can feel are out of his control, such as how others understand and react to stammering and how much stammering he is likely to experience in a given situation. Question 6 centres on the usefulness of the thought; that is, does it function to help the person in any way? Finally, question 8 asks the individual to consider the implications should a negative outcome result. For example, if a shop assistant does laugh when he asks for a sandwich, how bad would that be? What would be the implications? Would he still get the sandwich he wished to purchase?

84. NARRATIVE PRACTICE

i.   Background. Previously known as narrative therapy, narrative practice (NP) came out of the writings of Michael White and David Epston, principally in *Narrative Means to Therapeutic Ends* (1990), with additional material from the Dulwich Centre in Australia and others across the globe.

ii. Basic premise. NP has at its core the idea that a person constructs and gives meaning to his life through a series of stories or narratives he creates around lived experiences, as well as other tales given to him by family and society. For example, Cooper has a narrative of himself as a competitor running a race, constantly trying to keep up with others.

He also has a story, given to him by his parents, of a child who was gifted with lots of creative energy and enthusiasm for life. As his stories are unique to him, the individual is seen as the expert on his life. Neimeyer (1995) wrote:

> "as narrators, the significance of our lives is dictated by the stories that we live and that we tell – that is, by the ways that we link events in meaningful sequences and thereby constitute a sense of self as the protagonist of our own autobiography."
>
> (p. 22)

If a person has problem-based stories, such as those coloured by stammering experiences, then he can be helped through NP to deconstruct these accounts and reauthor a narrative which is stronger and less problem focused.

iii. Key components: NP delineates action and meaning or consciousness: action relates to specific behaviours, while consciousness is about emotions, thoughts, motivations, dreams and wishes. These two landscapes, as NP calls them, are interconnected. Bruner (2004) wrote:

> "There is a landscape of action on which events unfold . . . a second landscape of consciousness, the inner worlds of the protagonists involved in the action."
>
> (p. 698)

O'Dwyer and Ryan (2021) describe how NP works with these two landscapes belonging to a PWS:

> "NP uses this understanding of two landscapes to identify an action which resists or defies the problem story. The importance of this action is then acknowledged by connecting it to thoughts, emotions, dreams and ambitions preferred by the PWS and which provide a better fit to how he wants to see himself and live life."
>
> (p. 85)

iv. The processes involved in NP: The following are key processes:

- Externalisation of the problem. In this process, a person separates himself from the problem. As White and Epston (1990) wrote: 'the person is not the problem; the problem is the problem'. Thus, the client attending for speech and language therapy, is not 'a stammerer' but 'a person who stammers' or 'a person with a stammer'. At this stage, the PWS describes the problem and gives it a name. Next, he is invited to provide a rich description of how the problem is manifest and its effects, including examples from the past and present. This is followed by an evaluation of the problem by the individual, that is, is he content with the role it plays in his life? Finally, linking with his hopes and dreams, he reflects on his evaluation and considers new and different possibilities. O'Dwyer and Ryan (2021) provide a helpful list of questions which can be used in the externalisation process, including open questions, questions to gather information, clarification questions, examples of questions to ask about the person's evaluation of the problem and finally questions on his justification of his position. This final stage enables the person to thicken or deepen his commitment to his position.
- Identification of the unique outcome. This stage is concerned with identifying times when the problem is not as apparent or not as bad. As such, it has links with an aspect of solution-focused brief therapy (SFBT) (De Shazer 1985), in which there is a recognition of identifying 'exceptions' as part of the process of finding solutions to a problem. (See **Point 85**) Finding these exceptions or 'sparkling moments' is seen by O'Dwyer and Ryan (2021) as a 'turning point' in the therapy:

> "It is the entry point to the reauthoring process, the creation of an alternative story."

(p. 95)

The individual goes on to take a position on the unique outcome to decide if it connects with the values that are important to him and then determines the implications of the 'unique outcome' by deciding on future actions.

O'Dwyer and Ryan (2021) describe the structure of the conversation as:

- A rich description of the initiative or step taken
- Exploring the impact of this step on the person's relationships with himself and others
- Describing his experience of this step. 'Would you like more of this initiative?'
- 'Why take this position on it?'
- 'What does it tell others about what you value?'

(p. 95)

For example, Hadi decides to be open about his stammering. He elaborates with his therapist what this means in terms of his everyday activities: working as a bus driver, having conversations with travellers and work colleagues. When embarking on this change, he finds there is an impact on his relationships with some of his co-workers, especially those who have not heard him speaking in a non-fluent way. However, he is surprised at the lack of response and reaction from passengers asking for tickets. Following on from his experimentation with this change, he evaluates his experience and decides to continue with open stammering. Now that the appraisal of open stammering is positive, he reflects on how this influences the view of himself and the story he tells as a person who stammers.

- Reauthoring of the story. The following script is suggested to support inexperienced clinicians in starting a reauthoring conversation:

> "I want you to tell me a story. This story is about you and something you did or a time that you acted in a particular way that stands out to you. It might be that it appears to be different to the way you usually act."
>
> (O'Dwyer & Ryan 2021, p. 96)

There are four stages in the process of reauthoring, beginning with defining the 'unique outcome'. This is followed by mapping the effects of the exception in some possible situations, for example, 'When you did x or imagine yourself doing x, how did it feel to be doing that?' In the next stage, the person is asked to take a stance and evaluate the effects he has described, for example, 'Do you regard this as a positive or negative development in your life?' Finally, the clinician will invite her client to justify the evaluation he has given; again 'thickening' his commitment to his stance.

- Definitional ceremonies: White (2007) describes these ceremonies as rituals that:

> "provide people with the option of telling or performing the stories of their lives before an audience of carefully chosen outsider witnesses."
>
> (p. 165)

The definitional ceremony consists of four tellings of the person's story, with significant differences in the roles of the narrator and the listeners/audience.

- o The first account of the story involves the individual describing a significant event in their life story with invited outsider witness(es) acting as an audience.
- o Having listened to the story, the outsider witness then responds to what they have heard, with prompts from the therapist. The therapist asks questions of the person in the speaker/witness role around specific themes (White 2007), for example: Would you begin by talking about what you heard that you were most drawn to? (expression). What came to your mind while you were listening to this? (images). What is it about your own life that explains why you were drawn to these particular expressions? (resonance). Where did the story take you to in your mind as you listened? (transport). Thus, the witness individualises

the story, retelling it to the client, adding their own emphasis based on what they consider important features. Consequently, they present a retelling which adds insight to the original narrative.

- Following this outsider witness account of the story, the person then retells his story including the insights provided by the witness.
- Finally, facilitated by the clinician, the outsider witness and the individual engage in a discussion about their reflections on first three parts of the ceremony.

A detailed description and discussion of definitional ceremonies can be found in Leahy, O'Dwyer and Ryan (2012).

v. Advantages of using NP with a PWS: The use of NP when working with a PWS has been discussed by a number of writers (DiLollo et al. 2002; Logan 2013; O'Dwyer et al. 2018; O'Dwyer & Ryan 2021). DiLollo et al. (2002) list a number of benefits of using NP with a PWS:

- NP provides SLTs with an opportunity to better understand the role of stammering in the life of an PWS, how it affects his life and those around him
- NP provides an opportunity to explore the implications of 'stammerer' stereotypes about intelligence, emotional stability, honesty and competency and how these may affect the daily life of a PWS.
- NP provides an opportunity to address the impact of the self-description of 'I am a stammerer' on the process of speech and language therapy, which may aid a PWS in developing an understanding that such self-concepts may be detrimental to his progress in therapy and the long-term maintenance of therapeutically achieved changes.
- NP provides the opportunity to explore descriptions of self that are not subsumed by the description that stammering brings.
- NP provides an opportunity to explore the development of lifestyles that are preferred over a stammering lifestyle.

(p. 31)

85. SOLUTION-FOCUSED BRIEF THERAPY

i. Background. SFBT was developed out of clinical practice and is influenced by the philosophy of Wittgenstein and Buddhism. Because SBT is not based on a particular psychological theory, it cannot be regarded as a true psychological approach. However, it does contain a number of techniques which are relevant and useful when working with a PWS and merits inclusion here.

    SBFT emerged from the writings and clinical work of a psychiatrist and hypnotherapist, Milton Erickson. In the 1960s, a centre was establishing practising brief therapy, with practitioners Weakland, Watzlawick and Fisch at its heart. They developed the idea of reframing in which the issue or problem with which an individual might present was described in an alternative way in order for him to gain another perspective. There is evidence that this team worked with individuals who stammered (Watzlawick et al. 1974). Later a brief therapy centre was set up in Milwaukee led by Steve deShazer and his wife Kim Insoo Berg. Many of the components of SFBT arose from the writings and work of these two practitioners (De Shazer 1985, 1988).

ii. What is SFBT? SFBT is simply a way of talking to a client to enable him to change in the shortest possible time. (The average number of sessions is reported as between 2.7 and 5.5 [De Jong & Berg 2012]). However, it is not therapy done briefly. Rather, the change comes about by the individual elaborating on a description of his preferred future and the skills and resources he has to attain this outcome. He is also encouraged to provide examples from the past and present of instances when this preferred future has been realised.

    Interestingly, a practitioner using SFBT does not regard it as necessary for the person to describe his problem. In fact, she might actively steer the conversation to more solution talk (Berg & de Shazer 1993). Also, she will not give advice to her client, believing that it is more therapeutic for the individual to solve the issues himself.

"SFBT is a time-sensitive approach to exploring with clients how they would like their lives to be as a result of the therapy, and examining the skills and resources they have for getting there. It is not about the therapist assessing the type of problem the client has and/or providing the solution to the client's problem. It has to come from the client."

(Ratner et al. 2012, p. 4)

iii. Basic tenets of SFBT: SFBT is based on a number of principles:

- if it is not broken, don't fix it. Don't intervene when the problem is already solved, even though the person may not be aware of it
- look for exceptions. All problems have exceptions, that is, times when the problem is more or less absent. These times provide clues to finding a solution or solutions
- ask questions rather than telling clients what to do. SFBT makes questions the primary tool of communication and rarely makes direct challenges or confrontations to an individual
- the future is negotiated and created. The questions used in SFBT are almost always focused on the present and future. Therefore, rather than emphasising the past mistakes, the focus on solutions is believed to be more productive and empowering
- compliments. Compliments are another essential part of SFBT. Validating what the person already is doing well and acknowledging the magnitude of his problem encourages the individual to change while giving the message that the therapist understands and cares. Compliments in conversations can punctuate what he is doing right
- gentle nudging to do more of what is working. The SFBT therapist gently nudges the individual to do more of what has previously worked
- change is constant and inevitable. SFBT believes that stability in life is an illusion; life is constantly changing, and we are always changing. Noticing and paying

attention to small changes can set in motion more changes. The focus is on how to direct attention to more positive changes that are already happening

- the solution is not always directly related to the problem. This tenet seems to go against the intuition and knowledge about problems and solutions. According to the 'problem-solving' approach, there should be a logical and coherent relationship between problems and solutions. However, SFBT suggests being open to alternatives and the possibility of doing something differently.

Adapted from info@solutions-centre.org [accessed 24th June 2021].

iv. Key procedures of SFBT: There are a number of techniques which form the basis of SFBT sessions:

- problem-free talk. Usually at the beginning of a SFBT process, the clinician will facilitate a dialogue with her client talking about aspects of his life which do not involve the problem. This creates an opportunity to see the person holistically, not defined by his problem, and to notice any positive aspects: strengths and resources which may be referred to later in the process.
- goal development questions. In the first session(s), an individual would be asked a number of questions to describe his best hope for what will be different as a result of coming to therapy and what needs to happen as a result of coming. In this way, he will reflect that it was a good idea to attend the session and not a waste of his time.
- elaborating on the preferred future. Having identified the goal, the conversation then centres around generating a detailed description of what the person's life will look like once this goal has been achieved. This may include:
  ○ a 'Pre-Session Change Question', such as:

    Sometimes in between making an appointment and coming in, something happens to make things better. Did anything like that happen in your case?

If the individual says yes, then the clinician will ask follow-up questions and obtain details of how, when, and where things have improved and how this could continue.
○ the 'Miracle Question':

"Now, I want to ask you a strange question. Suppose that while you are sleeping tonight and the entire house is quiet, a miracle happens. The miracle is that the problem which brought you here is solved. However, because you are sleeping, you don't know that the miracle has happened. So, when you wake up tomorrow morning, what will be different that will tell you that a miracle has happened and the problem which brought you here is solved?"

(de Shazer 1988)

Follow-up questions after the miracle question are important to enable the person to elaborate on his description/imagining of the preferred future and its implications for his life. Examples include:

What will be the first thing you notice that would tell you that a miracle has happened, that things are different?

What would be the next thing you would notice while going about your day that would tell you the miracle has happened? (and the next . . .)

Who would be the first person to notice that things were different?

What might significant others notice (spouse, partner, parents, siblings, friends, work associates, peers etc.) that would tell them that the miracle has happened, that things are different or better?

Have there been times when you have seen pieces of this miracle happen?

○ Exceptions. Following on from the miracle question, the therapist will ask exception-finding questions. These are questions aimed at finding out about the occasions when the problem did not occur or was at its least troublesome:

"All problems have exceptions and paying attention to those times when exceptions occur is an important intervening tool since doing so indicates to the client that the therapist is confident of his ability to find solutions and that problems become more manageable when one has a clear sense of exceptions. Exceptions also point out what needs to be done to create badly needed solutions."

info@solutions-centre.org
[accessed 29th June 2021]

Examples of exception-finding questions include (for the sake of clarity, let us call the problem 'the elephant'):

Can you think back to a time when the elephant wasn't around? When was that? Tell me about that time?

Have there been times when you hardly noticed the elephant? When was that? Tell me about that time/those times.

Exceptions are viewed as 'little miracles'. It is important to:

o   identify them
o   explore them
o   extend their use and the frequency with which they occur
o   applaud and praise their occurrence.

• Scaling. The use of scale questions is possibly the most useful technique in the SFBT approach. Its flexibility allows it to be used to elicit and assess the efficacy of information on a scale from 0–10. It can be used to assess thoughts, feelings and behaviours and then facilitates the therapist and client together in determining the next stage in therapy.

Examples of scaling questions:

On a scale of 0–10, how big has the elephant been in your life?

On a scale of 0–10, what number would indicate to you that the elephant was not a problem anymore?

On a scale of 0–10, how big a problem is the elephant today?

What would have to happen to move how you rate the size of the elephant .5 or 1.0 down on the scale?

What would have to happen to keep that rating lower on the scale?

v. Using SFBT with a PWS. Turnbull and Stewart (2017) describe an instance when SFBT helped one of their clients:

"Looking to a preferred future helped George, a client who had had many years of therapy throughout his life, look at what he wanted and discover new ways in which he might achieve it. Using the 'miracle question' showed that what he wanted was to be more confident, assertive and less fearful of starting interactions. Looking at 'exceptions' showed him that there were indeed times when he was able to be all of these things, and 'scaling' helped him look at small stages to becoming how he wanted to be more often. He started to realise that, while he might always stammer, he did not have to let his stammer determine what sort of a person he was."

(p. 13)

REFERENCES

Andrade, C.R.F., Sassi, F.C., Juste, F.S. & Ercolin, B. (2008). Quality of life of individuals with persistent developmental stuttering. *Pro-Fono Scientific Update Magazine*, 20, 4, 219–224.

Blood, G. (1995). POWER: Relapse management with adolescents who stutter. *Language, Speech & Hearing Services in Schools*, 26, 169–180.

Bloodstein, O. & Bernstein Ratner, N. (2008). *A Handbook on Stuttering*, 6th edition. Clifton Park, NY: Thomson Delmar Learning.

Cooper, E.H. & Cooper, C.S. (1995). Treating fluency disordered adolescents. *Journal of Communication Disorders*, 28, 125–142.

Corcoran, J.A. & Stewart, M. (1998). Stories of stuttering: A qualitative analysis of interview narratives. *Journal of Fluency Disorders*, 23, 247–264.

Craig, A., Blumgart, E. & Tran, Y. (2009). The impact of stuttering on the quality of life in adult people who stutter. *Journal of Fluency Disorders*, 34, 61–71.

Craig, A. & Tran, Y. (2006). Chronic and social anxiety in people who stutter. *Advances in Psychiatric Treatment*, 12, 63–68.

Crichton-Smith, I. (2002). Communicating in the real world: Accounts from people who stammer. *Journal of Fluency Disorders*, 27, 333–352.

Daly, D., Simon, C.A. & Burnett-Stolnack, M. (1995). Helping adolescents who stutter focus on fluency. *Language, Speech & Hearing Services in Schools*, 26, 162–168.

Everard, R. (2019). Making a difference: Developing the evidence base for stammering modification. *Signal*, 52, 16–17.

Klompas, M. & Ross, E. (2004). Life experiences of people who stutter, and the perceived impact of stuttering on quality of life: Personal accounts of South African individuals. *Journal of Fluency Disorders*, 29, 4, 275–305.

Koedoot, C., Bouwmans, C., Franken, M.C. & Stolk, E. (2011). Quality of life in adults who stutter. *Journal of Communication Disorders*, 44, 4, 429–43.

Menzies, R., Onslow, M. & Packman, A. (1999). Anxiety and stuttering: Exploring a complex relationship. *American Journal of Speech & Language Pathology*, 8, 1, 3–10.

Van Riper, C. (1973). *The Treatment of Stuttering*. Englewood Cliffs, NJ: Prentice-Hall, Inc.

Watson, J. (1995). Exploring the attitudes of adults who stutter. *Journal of Communication Disorders*, 28, 143–164.

Williams, D. (1957). A point of view about 'stuttering'. *Journal of Speech & Hearing Disorders*, 22, 3, 390–397.

MINDFULNESS

Baer, R.A., Smith, G.T. & Allen, K.B. (2004). Assessment of mindfulness by self-report: *The Kentucky Inventory of Mindfulness Skills Assessment*, 11, 191–206.

Boyle, M.P. (2011). Mindfulness training in stuttering therapy: A tutorial for speech-language pathologists. *Journal of Fluency Disorders*, 36, 2, 122–129.

Brocklehurst, P. Mindfulness and stuttering: How can mindfulness help? www.stammeringresearch.org/mindfulness.pdf [Accessed May 2021].

Cheasman, C. (2013). A mindful approach to stammering. In C. Cheasman, R. Everard & S. Simpson (eds.), *Stammering Therapy from the Inside*. Guildford: J & R Press.

Cheasman, C. (2021). Integrating mindfulness into therapy with people who stammer. In T. Stewart (ed.), *Stammering Resources for Adults and Teenagers: Integrating New Evidence into Clinical Practice*. London: Routledge, Taylor & Francis Group.

Fairburn, C.G., Cooper, Z., De Veer, S., Brouwers, A., Evers, W. & Tomik, W. (2009). A pilot study of the psychological impact of the mindfulness-based stress reduction program on persons who stutter. *European Psychotherapy*, 9, 39–56.

Kabat-Zinn, J. (1994). *Wherever You Go, There You Are*. New York: Hyperion.

Kabat-Zinn, J. (2005). *Coming to Our Senses*. New York: Hyperion.

Segal, Z.V., Williams, J.M.G. & Teasdale, J.D. (2002). *Mindfulness Based Cognitive Therapy for Depression: A New Approach to Preventing Relapse*. New York: Guilford.

OTHER RESOURCES

Cheasman, C. Mindfulness and its relevance to stammering – City Lit London UK National Centre for Work with Adults Who Stammer. www.ecsf.eu/userfiles/files/Cheasman.

Silverman, E.M. (2012). *Mindfulness & Stuttering: Using Eastern Strategies to Speak with Greater Ease.* North Charleston, SC: CreateSpace. www.stutteringtreatment. org/blog/mindfulness-for-people-who-stutter-4-guided-meditations.

ACCEPTANCE AND COMMITMENT THERAPY

Beilby, J.M. & Byrnes, M.L. (2010a). *Effectiveness of a Mindfulness-Based Acceptance and Commitment Therapy to Improve Quality of Life of Adults Who Stutter.* Presentation at the European Symposium of Fluency Disorders Antwerp, Belgium.

Beilby, J.M. & Byrnes, M.L. (2010b). *Evaluation of the Effectiveness of a Mindfulness and Acceptance Group Program to Improve Communication Fears, Experiential Avoidance and Quality of Life of Adults Who Stutter.* Presentation at the Speech Pathology Australia National Conference, Melbourne, Australia.

Beilby, J.M. & Byrnes, M.L. (2012). Acceptance and commitment therapy for people who stutter. *Perspectives on Fluency and Fluency Disorders,* 22, 1, 34–46.

Beilby, J.M., Byrnes, M.L. & Yaruss, J.S. (2012). Acceptance and commitment therapy for adults who stutter: Psychosocial adjustment and speech fluency. *Journal of Fluency Disorders,* 37, 289–299.

Byrnes, M., Hart, M., Beilby, J., Blacker, D. & Schug, S. (2010). *Effectiveness of Acceptance and Commitment Therapy Group Program for Individuals Post Spinal Cord Injury and Stroke and People Who Stutter: Similarities and Differences.* Presentation at the 4th Australian & New Zealand Conference` of Acceptance and Commitment Therapy South Australia, Australia.

Cheasman, C. (2021). Integrating mindfulness into therapy with people who stammer. In T. Stewart (ed.), *Stammering Resources for Adults and Teenagers: Integrating New Evidence into Clinical Practice.* London: Routledge, Taylor & Francis Group.

Everard, R. & Cheasman, C. (2021). Integrating ACT into stammering therapy. In T. Stewart (ed.), *Stammering Resources for Adults & Teenagers: Integrating New Evidence into Clinical Practice*. London: Routledge, Taylor & Francis Group.

Flaxman, P.E., McIntosh, R. & Oliver, J. (2019). *Acceptance and Commitment Training (ACT) for Workplace Settings: Trainer Manual*. London: University of London.

Harris, R. (2009). *ACT Made Simple*. Oakland, CA: New Harbinger Publications Inc.

Plexico, L., Manning, W.H. & Di Lollo, A. (2005). A phenomenological understanding of successful stuttering management. *Journal of Fluency Disorders*, 30, 1, 1–22.

Plexico, L., Manning, W.H. & Levitt, H. (2009). Coping responses by adults who stutter: II. Approaching the problem and achieving agency. *Journal of Fluency Disorders*, 34, 108–126.

Yaruss, Y. (2012). What does it mean to say that a person 'accepts' stuttering? In P. Reitzes & D. Reitzes (eds.), *Stuttering: Inspiring Stories & Professional Wisdom*. Chapel Hill, NC: StutterTalk Publication No 1.

OTHER RESOURCES

Cheasman, C., Simpson, S. & Everard, R. (2015). Acceptance and speech work: The challenge. Presentation at the 10th Oxford Dysfluency Conference, Oxford. *Procedia – Social and Behavioral Sciences*, 193, 72–81.

Tyndall, I. Growing a beautiful new shell for all to see. *Stamma website British Stammering Association* [Accessed May 2021].

www.actmindfully.com.au

www.thehappinesstrap.com

PERSONAL CONSTRUCT PSYCHOLOGY AND THERAPY

Dalton, P. (1983). Psychological approaches to the treatment of stuttering. In P. Dalton (ed.), *Approaches to the Treatment of Stuttering*. London: Croom Helm.

Dalton, P. (1994). *Counselling People with Communication Problems*. London: Sage Publications.

DiLollo, A., Neimeyer, R. & Manning, W. (2002). A personal construct psychology view of relapse: Indications for a narrative therapy component to stuttering treatment. *Journal of Fluency Disorders*, 27, 1, 19–42.

Evesham, M. & Fransella, F. (1985). Stuttering relapse: The effect of a combined speech and psychological reconstruction programme. *British Journal of Disorders of Communication*, 20, 237–248.

Evesham, M. & Huddleston, A. (1983). Teaching stutterers the skill of fluent speech as a preliminary to the study of relapse. *British Journal of Disorders of Communication*, 18, 31–38.

Fransella, F. (1972). *Personal Change and Reconstruction*. London: Academic Press.

Fransella, F. & Dalton, P. (1990). *Personal Construct Counselling in Action*. London: Sage Publications.

Hayhow, R. & Levy, C. (1989). *Working with Stuttering*. Bicester, UK: Winslow Press.

Kelly, G.A. (1955). *The Psychology of Personal Constructs: Vol. 1*. New York: Norton.

Stewart, T. (1996). Good maintainers and poor maintainers: A personal construct approach to an old problem. *Journal of Fluency Disorders*, 21, 22–48.

Stewart, T. & Birdsall, M. (2001). A review of the contribution of personal construct psychology to stammering therapy. *Journal of Constructivist Psychology*, 14, 215–226.

Stewart, T. & Brosh, H. (1997). The use of drawings in the management of adults who stammer. *Journal of Fluency Disorders*, 22, 1, 35–50.

Williams, R. (1995). Personal construct theory in use with people who stutter. In M. Fawcus (ed.), *Stuttering from Theory to Practice*. London: Whurr Publishers.

COGNITIVE BEHAVIOURAL THERAPY

Andrew, G. & Craig, A. (1982). Stuttering: Overt and covert assessment of the speech of treated subjects. *Journal of Speech and Hearing Disorders*, 47, 96–99.

Bennet-Levy, J., Westbrook, D., Fennell, M., Cooper, M., Rouf, K. & Hackman, A. (2004). Behavioural experiments: Historical and conceptual underpinnings. In J. Bennett-Levy, G. Butler, M. Fennell, A. Hackman, M. Mueller & D. Westbrook (eds.), *Oxford Guide to Behavioural Experiments in Cognitive Therapy*. Oxford: Oxford University Press.

Blood, G.W. (1995). A behavioral-cognitive therapy program for adults who stutter: Computers and counseling. *Journal of Communication Disorders*, 28, 2, 165–180.

Craig, A. & Andrews, G. (1985). The prediction and prevention of relapse in stuttering. The value of self-control techniques and locus of control measures. *Behavior Modification*, 9, 427–442.

Craig, A. & Tran, Y. (2006). Chronic and social anxiety in people who stutter. *Advances in Psychiatric Treatment*, 12, 63–68.

Howie, P.M., Tanner, S. & Andrews, G. (1981). Short and long term outcomes in an intensive treatment program for adult stutterers. *Journal of Speech & Hearing Disorders*, 46, 104–109.

Iverach, L., Rapee, R.M., Wong, Q.J.J. & Lowe, R. (2017). Maintenance of social anxiety in stuttering: A cognitive-behavioral model. *American Journal of Speech-Language Pathology*, 26, 2, 540–556.

Langevin, M., Huinck, W., Kully, D., Peters, H., Lomheim, H. & Tellers, M. (2006). A cross-cultural, long-term outcome evaluation of the ISTAR Comprehensive Stuttering Program across Dutch and Canadian adults who stutter. *Journal of Fluency Disorders*, 31, 229–56.

Maxwell, D. (1982). Cognitive and behavioral self-control strategies: Applications for the clinical management of adult stutterers. *Journal of Fluency Disorders*, 7, 403–432.

Menzies, R.G., O'Brian, S., Onslow, M., Packman, A., St Clare, T. & Block, S. (2008). An experimental clinical trial of a cognitive-behavior therapy package for chronic stuttering. *Journal of Speech Language, & Hearing Research*, 51, 6, 1451.

Menzies, R.G., Onslow, M., Packman, A. & O'Brian, S. (2009). Cognitive behavior therapy for adults who stutter: A tutorial for speech-language pathologists. *Journal of Fluency Disorders*, 34, 187–200.

Plexico, L., Manning, W.H. & Di Lollo, A. (2005). A phenomenological understanding of successful stuttering management. *Journal of Fluency Disorders*, 30, 1, 1–22.

St Clare, T., Menzies, R.G., Onslow, M., Packman, A., Thompson, R. & Block, S. (2009). Unhelpful thoughts and beliefs linked to social anxiety in stuttering: Development of a measure. *International Journal of Language & Communication Disorders*, 44, 3, 338–351.

Turnbull, J. & Stewart, T. (2017). *The Dysfluency Resource Book*, 2nd edition. London: Routledge, Taylor & Francis Group.

OTHER RESOURCES

Butler, G. & Hope, T. (1995). *Manage Your Mind: The Mental Fitness Guide*. Oxford: Oxford University Press.

NARRATIVE PRACTICE

Bruner, J.S. (2004). Life as narrative. *Social Research*, 71, 1, 691–711.

De Shazer, S. (1985). *Keys to Solution in Brief Therapy*. New York: Norton.

DiLollo, A., Neimeyer, R. & Manning, W. (2002). A personal construct psychology view of relapse: Indications for a narrative therapy component to stuttering treatment. *Journal of Fluency Disorders*, 27, 1, 19–42.

Leahy, M.M., O'Dwyer, M. & Ryan, F. (2012). Witnessing stories: Definitional ceremonies in narrative therapy with adults who stutter. *Journal of Fluency Disorders*, 37, 4, 234–241.

Logan, J. (2013). New stories of stammering: A narrative approach. In C. Cheasman, R. Everard & S. Simpson (eds.), *Stammering Therapy from the Inside: New Perspectives on Working with Young People and Adults*. Guildford: J & R Press Ltd.

Neimeyer, R.A. (1995). Constructivist psychotherapies: Features, foundations, and future directions. In R.A. Neimeyer & R.J. Mahoney (eds.), *Constructivism in Psychotherapy*. Washington, DC: American Psychological Association.

O'Dwyer, M. & Ryan, F. (2021). Narrative practice: Identifying and changing problem stories about stammering. In T. Stewart (ed.), *Stammering Resources for Adults and Teenagers: Integrating New Evidence into Clinical Practice*. London: Routledge, Taylor & Francis Group.

O'Dwyer, M., Walsh, I.P. & Leahy, M.M. (2018). The role of narratives in the development of stuttering. *American Journal of Speech & Language Pathology*, 27, 3, 1164–1179.

White, M. (2007). *Maps of Narrative Practice*. New York: Norton.

White, M. & Epston, D. (1990). *Narrative Means to Therapeutic Ends*. New York: Norton.

OTHER RESOURCES

https://dulwichcentre.com.au/. This is the website for The Dulwich Center in Adelaide Australia, founded by Michael White. The website includes resources and free online training.

Morgan, A. (2000). *What Is Narrative Therapy?* Adelaide: Dulwich Centre Publications.

Ryan, F. (2018). *Stories from the Other Side: Outcomes from Narrative Therapy for People Who Stutter*. Unpublished thesis.

SOLUTION-FOCUSED BRIEF THERAPY

Berg, I.K. & de Shazer, S. (1993). Making numbers talk: Language in therapy. In S. Friedman (ed.), *The New Language of Change: Constructive Collaboration in Psychotherapy*. New York: Guilford Press.

De Jong, P. & Berg, K.I. (2012). *Interviewing for Solutions*, 4th edition. Belmont, CA: Cengage Learning, Brooks/Cole.

De Shazer, S. (1985). *Keys to Solution in Brief Therapy*. New York: Norton.

De Shazer, S. (1988). *Clues: Investigating Solutions in Brief Therapy*. New York: Norton.

Ratner, H., George, E. & Iveson, C. (2012). *Solution Focused Brief Therapy: 100 Key Points & Techniques*. London: Routledge, Taylor & Francis Group.

Watzlawick, P., Weakland, J.H. & Fisch, R. (1974). *Change: Principles of Problem Formation and Problem Solution*. New York: Norton.

OTHER RESOURCES

Burns, K. (2006). *Focus on Solutions: A Health Professional's Guide*. London: Wiley. info@solutions-centre.org.

De Shazer, S. (1994). *Words Were Originally Magic*. New York: Norton.

Section J

MAINTAINING POSITIVE OUTCOMES AND PLANNING FOR THE RE-EMERGENCE OF ROLES AND BEHAVIOURS

(Note: I considered writing this section as another component of Therapy [see **Section E**] but decided to give it due weight, as it is one of the most important phases of change.)

86. DEFINING THIS STAGE

Most authors would define this stage as relapse. However, I have tried to avoid the use of medical terminology in this text, and relapse has certain medical connotations. This stage for a PWS can take many forms and involve cognitive, affective and behavioural departures from what has been achieved. It can range from brief periods to longer periods, which often result in frustration and more significant affective reactions.

87. HOW CAN SUCH A PERIOD OF DIFFICULTY BE IDENTIFIED?

Is there a period beyond which the PWS cannot get back his previous gains? Identifying a period when setbacks occur is best done by the PWS himself and will be based on his awareness and the degree of difference between his current well-being when compared to a previous or desired state.

88. BACKGROUND

It is difficult to quantify the number of individuals who stammer who experience returns to previous states following a therapeutic intervention (Craig 1998). Different estimates have been reported in the literature, ranging from 23% (Boberg & Kully 1994) 30–60% (Howie et al. 1981) when objective assessments were used and 73% based on self-report (Craig & Hancock 1995). The accuracy of the reporting is confused by the cyclical nature of these stages. In a study of 109 adults who stammered, the mean number of setbacks was reported to be three per year, with the occurrences lasting from one week to five months (Craig & Hancock 1995).

The key point here is that such times are to be expected. Van Riper wrote:

"Relapses and remissions are the rule, not the exception."
(p. 178)

It occurs normally when a person is engaged in a process of change. Therefore, it should be planned and managed in a therapeutic journey.

89. MAINTENANCE AND ITS PLACE IN THERAPY

When structuring his therapy, Van Riper (1973) divided his engagement with a PWS into a sequence of phases consisting of:

- Identification
- Desensitization
- Modification
- Stabilization

(p. 205)

The last phase, also referred to as maintenance, Van Riper believed to be necessary in order for a person to manage the strength of his avoidance and struggle reactions, which are 'remarkably resistant to complete extinction' (p. 350). While Van Riper's primary objectives of this phase were the maintenance of fluency gains, he also referred to the need to manage the self-concept of the PWS and the reactions of others to the changes that have been made. Included in the activities of the stabilisation phase were:

- a review of therapy and the progress made
- PWS kept a diary/log of experiences
- PWS described hypothetical problems and their solutions
- activities designed to 'buffer' or toughen resistance to negative listener reactions
- development of positive thinking
- reconstruction of self in speaker role
- shift of PWS into being his own therapist
- formal ending of therapy.

90. INTEGRATION OF STRATEGIES TO MANAGE SETBACKS IN THERAPY

The situation has moved on considerably from the procedures described previously. Difficulties in maintenance are accepted as a normal part of the change process, and therefore contingencies (including those listed by Van Riper) are constantly worked on throughout therapy.

From the first session, I suggest the individual has a special notebook or note page on his phone/tablet to record those pieces of information or ideas he believes are important to maintain his desired outcomes. This process is relevant to any change, irrespective of the nature of the therapy approach which is being embarked upon, that is, 'stammer more easily', 'speak more fluently', 'stammer more proudly' or psychological change.

91. WHAT DOES A PWS NEED TO BE ABLE TO MAINTAIN HIS THERAPY GAINS?

In a qualitative study, Plexico et al. (2005) interviewed seven PWS to explore their experience of stammering and the process of change. The individual interview transcriptions were analysed for themes relating to successful and unsuccessful management of stammering. The themes pertaining to successful management were:

- continued management
- self-acceptance and fear reduction
- unrestricted interactions
- sense of freedom
- optimism.

> "Successful management of stuttering is characterized by an optimistic and positive interpretation of life. In spite of the fact that self-management of stuttering continues, the possibility of stuttering is no longer a major theme. There is a sense of appreciation for what has been accomplished . . . more dominant themes indicate that life choices are no longer restricted by anxiety or fear associated with stuttering or the possibility of stuttering. There is an obvious sense of freedom to act and speak on one's own behalf."
>
> (p. 16)

92. STRATEGIES FOR MAINTENANCE

As a PWS works through his therapy process, he collects the strategies or tools he needs to maintain his desired outcomes. At each stage, there are skills he may incorporate in his toolbox. For example, in **identification** (see **Section G, Point 63**), he could have developed the ability to monitor specific aspects of speech and/or features of his lifestyle which can give rise to struggle (e.g. levels of stress, poor sleep). In desensitisation activities (see **Section E, Point 49**), he may have found benefits in being open with friends and work colleagues about stammering. Consequently, he will include in his tool box the need to mention his stammer periodically in conversations as an important strategy. In addition, he could decide to add ways of expressing himself assertively in specific situations, having discovered this to be useful to advocate stammering (see **Section E, Point 48** and **Section H, Point 75**) with others.

i.   Aims: The aim is for each individual to develop a unique set of strategies, tailor-made to his needs, set of circumstances and anticipated issues, which he is able to take forward once therapy comes to an end. Ideally the strategies should be dynamic rather than prescribed. For example, having a problem-solving or solution-focused approach is preferable rather than a set of behaviours for each specific problem. The tools should also reflect an holistic approach to maintenance and as such include the management of cognitions, emotions and behaviours.

ii. What to include: Writing a toolbox can be a difficult task for some, and the PWS may feel a little overwhelmed by the comprehensive nature and level of detail required. To support his process of writing, he can be given examples of toolboxes written by previous clients (anonymised, of course). Alternatively, the therapist can provide a list of headings as guidance. For example:

*   daily tools
*   weekly tools
*   occasional tools
*   tools to practise
*   tools for specific situations.

Or a more detailed template may be used by a PWS. An example is given in the following:

A Template for Developing a Tool Box

Tools	Behaviours	Emotions	Thoughts
Everyday			
Weekly			
Occasionally			
Regular practice			
To do when things are going well			
To do when things are going less well			
Specific situation practice			
Enlisting the help of others			
Other			

(Based on Turnbull & Stewart 2017)

Emma, a client, developed her own format, which proved valuable for her ongoing maintenance, which is summarised in the following table. A full version can be found in Turnbull and Stewart (2017).

Sample of Emma's toolbox taken from Handout 47, p. 201, Turnbull & Stewart 2017

EMMA'S TOOLBOX			
	GOOD DAY	EVERY DAY	BAD DAY
EYE CONTACT	*Keep eye contact when I stammer with unfamiliar people*	*Good eye contact when I initiate & during interactions*	*Remember to give it to them, bam smack between the eyes!*
RELAXATION	*Pause*	*Collect thoughts*	*3-minute breathing space*
SELF-ADVERTISING	*All the time – out & proud!*	*Introductions: introduce stammer first then name*	*Use support network – talk about it*
POSITIVE COGNITIONS	*Tackle unsupportive thoughts*	*Replace unhelpful thoughts with more supportive ones*	*Think: is there anything else that is contributing to the way I feel? Be objective, cut self some slack!*

In addition to this 'good day, every day, bad day' plan, Emma also included a practice plan and notes on handling some specific situations (e.g. phone calls) in her extensive and well-prepared tool box.

93. ENDINGS

Once the tool box has been written, it can be used to mark a rite of passage out of therapy. The PWS can read it aloud to the therapist and/or to a group of clients (if he is involved in group therapy). It is also an opportunity to invite others, such as SOs to witness and hear the account of future strategies, some of which may carry some consequences for them (i.e. require some input or support). Finally, the transcript provides the clinician with a useful summary in the PWS's own words of what he believes has been achieved in therapy and is carrying away with him. It can then be used, once permission is given by the person, as an example to show others and, when appropriate, may form the basis for any review appointments with the individual in the future.

REFERENCES

Boberg, E. & Kully, D. (1994). Long-term results of an intensive treatment program for adults and adolescents who stutter. *Journal of Speech & Hearing Research*, 37, 1050–1059.

Craig, A.R. (1998). Relapse following treatment for stuttering: A critical review and correlative data. *Journal of Fluency Disorders*, 23, 1–30.

Craig, A.R. & Hancock, K. (1995). Self-reported factors related to relapse following treatment for stuttering. *Australian Journal of Human Communication Disorders*, 23, 48–60.

Howie, P.M., Tanner, S. & Andrews, G. (1981). Short- and long-term outcomes in an intensive treatment program for adult stutterers. *Journal of Speech & Hearing Disorders*, 46, 104–109.

Plexico, L., Manning, W.H. & DiLollo, A. (2005). A phenomenological understanding of successful stuttering management. *Journal of Fluency Disorders*, 30, 1–22.

Turnbull, J. & Stewart, T. (2017). *The Dysfluency Resource Book*, 2nd edition. London: Routledge, Taylor & Francis Group.

Van Riper, C. (1973). *The Treatment of Stuttering*. Englewood Cliffs, NJ: Prentice-Hall, Inc.

Section K

SUPPORT NETWORKS

94. THE CONTEXT

Stammering does not happen in isolation, nor are the ramifications purely felt by the speaker. The PWS is part of a network of family, possibly including siblings, partners, children, friends, peers and others. His stammering will occur in social interactions with these individuals. Consequently, those others, significant in the life of the PWS, are likely to be implicated in his change process and effected in some way by stammering and the PWS's emotional and cognitive responses to it.

95. SIGNIFICANT OTHERS AS AGENTS OF CHANGE

There is much evidence regarding the important role an SO has in a person's therapeutic process. Boberg and Kully (1985) identified the vital role a spouse plays as an

> I wish I had realised how much family/partners etc play a major role in therapy.
> Jeanette Zammit (Personal Communication 2021)

agent for change when he/she is engaged in therapy. Boberg and Boberg (1990) also found that the active involvement of partners in therapy enabled a PWS to achieve greater success than would have normally occurred. Corcoran and Stewart (1998) showed that supportive relationships were beneficial to the overall experience of therapy. Also, in conversations with a PWS and their partner, the partner was shown to be the primary facilitator, crucial in ensuring the success of the interactions (Hughes et al. 2010).

DOI: 10.4324/9781003177890-12

Finally, what of the children in a family where a family member is a PWS? Boberg and Boberg demonstrated the positive results of being open about stammering with *all* family members, including the children, rather than perpetuating a 'conspiracy of silence' regarding stammering. There were demonstrable benefits in having the children involved in therapy in some way (e.g. as critical observers, conversational partners).

All of this evidence points to the importance of involving SOs in the therapeutic process of a PWS.

96. THE NATURE OF SO INVOLVEMENT IN THERAPY

As previously stated, a key message for therapists who are unsure of how best to help a client in a specific situation is to ASK THE PWS. In terms of establishing how their individual PWS would like to be supported by his SO, the therapist will engage in a detailed conversation with him and construct the support around his stated preferences.

> I would have liked to know if it was useful and/or necessary to involve family members in the treatment of stuttering.
> Jo Van der Sypt (Personal Communication 2021)

For example, research (Hughes 2007) in which PWS were asked about the support they received from their families indicates that there was a significant amount of what is termed 'surface' support. However, in this study, many individuals reported wanting different support. They wished to discuss stammering openly in the family, especially the emotional aspects. Where they were engaged in therapy, they also wanted that to be the subject of conversations between the PWS and family members.

> "Participants desired for family members to understand their needs and approach them regarding the topic of stuttering. Finally, participants felt it was important for family members to learn how to listen to

them, and to discuss the feelings that were associated with stuttering."

(p. 28)

It is therefore clear that a number of actions are needed in a therapy process to ensure that SOs are appropriately involved. Following on from establishing the nature of change and the stated goals of the PWS, the therapist will:

- discuss with the PWS which SO(s) he would wish to include in the therapy process and how this will take place.
- the relevant SO(s) will be invited to a meeting with the PWS and therapist will i) outline the goals of therapy and the specific implications of change and ii) discuss the involvement of the SO(s) in the therapy process. A follow-up discussion may be arranged if and when required. (A therapist may consider carrying out a home visit where several family members and children are to be included in the process. It can be more relaxed for the family and valuable for the clinician to see the PWS's context for therapy.)
- periodic review meetings will be planned and put in diaries for progress to be appraised, any difficulties subjected to a problem-solving or solution-focused approach and positive outcomes validated.
- in a group therapy context, an open invitation for SO(s) to attend at their convenience may be considered by the group. Alternatively, specific sessions to include SOs can be arranged at regular intervals and relevant activities planned for these sessions. An example of such a session is given in Turnbull and Stewart (2017), who describe an activity in which the SOs and group members discuss their collective understanding of some statements based on Sheehan's approach-avoidance theory. For example:
    - What you call your stammering consists mostly of the tricks and strategies you use to cover it up. It is far better to stammer openly and honestly than it is to use a trick, even if it is temporarily successful.

- In accepting yourself as a person who has a stammer, you choose the route to becoming a more honest, relaxed speaker. The more you run away from your stammering, the more you will stammer. The more you are open and courageous, the more you will develop good communication.

(p. 216)

In all communications with SOs, it is crucial to maintain transparency and avoid any return to the conspiracy of silence. Thus, all conversations, emails, telephone calls and so on between the clinician and SOs will involve the PWS and/or be reported to him.

97. THE OTHER SIDE OF STAMMERING

How does stammering impact the significant others of a PWS? In one of the first studies in this area, Boberg and Boberg (1990) studied how the spouse of a PWS was affected by their partner's stammering. A number of issues were identified, including the emotional effects of the stammer and anxieties that were prevalent before marriage and present specifically on their wedding day.

Using questions adapted from Boberg and Boberg's (1990) interview protocol, Beilby et al. (2013) studied 20 working couples whose ages ranged from 20s to 60s, some with children, some with no children and a number of grandparents. Their stated aims were:

"(a) to investigate what personal experiences and themes exist for both members of a couple dyad when one member of the couple stutters and (b) to examine whether the partners have different experiences with respect to the impact of stuttering on their lives."

(p. 14)

The key findings have important implications for clinical practice:

- PWS and partners report congruence in the way they view stammering, that is, their knowledge of, personal reactions to and the effects of stammering on communication

- participants shared life experiences regarding reactions to stammering. Nearly half of the partners expressed feelings of 'overprotection' and 'anguish' while watching the PWS speak
- the couples referred to 'acceptance' of stammering while not regarding this as a limitation in their relationship
- honesty and integrity were discussed by couples as important features of their relationship
- the comments of the spouses reflected the intricate and complex changes brought about by therapy
- partners described the type of support they provided. This ranged from providing a target word in a conversation to patiently waiting for the PWS to express himself without pressure.

Linn and Caruso (1998) cite Rolland (1994) when proposing stammering acts like a chronic disorder, becoming a third member of a close relationship. Consequently, stammering can impact routine activities, for example, influencing decisions about who orders in restaurants/cafes, who answers the land-line and who talks to the neighbours. A PWS who is progressing in therapy may decide he wants and is able to take on actions he has shied away from in the past. This will disturb the balance in a relationship that has operated on established tacit roles for a number of years. For example, as Ethan became more confident in his communication, he started ordering his own choices in restaurants and making his own phone calls. This came as a surprise to his partner, and she felt her role with him under threat, as she had previously done all these things for him. It is therefore essential that the change and the implications of the change be discussed at the outset and ongoing conversations regarding the impact on a dyad and roles with other SOs be carried out at regular intervals during therapy.

> "In discussing issues . . . particularly stuttering, a couple's relationship becomes stronger through communication, understanding and the building of trust."
> (Linn & Caruso 1998, p. 14)

Case: Mitch, a construction worker in his 40s, referred himself for therapy. He had a mild overt stammer, with some sound and word repetitions and fillers, such as 'you know', 'erm'. However, he had significant covert components to his stammer, including levels of avoidance which affected every aspect of his interactions on a daily basis. For example:

- using stalling or delaying tactics, e.g. pretending to have forgotten, asking his conversational partner to repeat what they had said to stall for time, using starter phrases, coughing, laughing, clearing his throat, sniffing, snorting
- linguistic gymnastics, e.g. changing words, changing sentence order, using circumlocution
- using distraction techniques, e.g. pinching himself, swearing, raising the volume of his voice, writing and speaking simultaneously
- having specific strategies for managing certain situations, e.g. while on the mobile phone blaming the signal when he is having a silent block, walking away from a shop counter or takeaway if there is a queue and ordering the drink that is most difficult to say first at the bar.

However, the biggest avoidance was that he had not told his wife of 20 years, or teenage daughter, about his stammer. He had numerous behaviours to manage this secret, and coming to therapy became part of that list.

Finally in one group therapy session, when SOs had been invited to attend (Mitch, of course, did not bring anyone), he observed the various ways that other group members were supported by their SOs. This came as a revelation to him, and he realised for the first time how his avoidance enabled his feelings of isolation and separation.

After the group, Mitch decided to take his wife out to dinner and make her aware of everything. (He had begun the process by declaring that he had 'something important to tell' her. Goodness knows what she anticipated!)

As a therapist, I had enormous concerns about what this revelation would do to a relationship founded on a role which was about to be revealed as false. Mitch was not the angry, blaspheming, easily irritated, loud person he portrayed. Rather he was anxious, wary, deeply afraid, vulnerable and needing understanding and support.

In this instance, the stammer was a silent third partner; affecting how interactions in daily situations played out. In the end, the relationship proved to be made of strong stuff; Mitch's wife, while previously totally unaware of his stammer, listened and heard this new story and fully embraced her redefined role as supporter in his journey to find his different self.

98. SUPPORT GROUPS

Support groups in this context are also known as self-help or advocacy groups and include face-to-face meetings of PWS, online groups with zoom meetings and chat rooms.

i.   The importance of support groups: these meetings have been found to play an important part specifically in therapy (Klassen & Kroll 2005) and more generally in the 'successful management' of stammering. (Plexico et al. 2005).

What support groups provide: In my clinical experience, I have found that groups provide empathy, encouragement, motivation and a sense of community. The research reflects the numerous benefits for a PWS of membership of such groups:

* Plexico et al. (2005) found that participants in their study (who were PWS) stated that:

"the support systems provided them with the chance to connect with others who stuttered, disclose their stuttering, and exchange information about stuttering."
(p. 11)

* Manning (2001) highlighted:
    ○   reduced isolation:
        Possibly for the first time in his life, the person will find that he is among many others who share a common problem. He finds that the unique part of him that has,

for so long, set him apart from others now provides a
way to connect and bond with many people.

(p. 430)

- o Opportunities to practice strategies and stabilise
    cognitive changes following treatment (p. 431)
- o Facilitation of personal change, . . . provision of
    information and advice and discussion of alterna-
    tive treatments, fundraising and political activities
    relating to the goals of the group (p. 431)
- o providing 'an effective voice for improved training
    and service delivery to professional and legislative
    groups' (p. 433).
- Boyle (2013), in his study, reported:

    "Participants with support group experience as a
    whole demonstrated lower internalized stigma, were
    more likely to believe that they would stutter for the
    rest of their lives, and less likely to perceive production
    of fluent speech as being highly or moderately important
    when talking to other people, compared to participants
    with no support group experience. Individuals who
    joined support groups to help others feel better about
    themselves reported higher self-esteem, self-efficacy,
    and life satisfaction, and lower internalized stigma and
    perceived stuttering severity, compared to participants
    with no support group experience."

    He concluded that his findings:

    "support the notion that self-help support groups
    limit internalization of negative attitudes about the
    self, and that focusing on helping others feel better in a
    support group context is linked to higher levels of psy-
    chological well-being."

    (p. 368)

- Liddle and Adams (2021), in their chapter on working
    with self-help groups, write of the different possibilities

self-help groups provide when compared to the therapy alternative:

"they tend to be run more flexibly than professional services. This can create more opportunities for a wider range of activities and experiences and can allow groups the freedom to function in ways that benefit participants."

(p. 215)

In addition, they discuss the function of a self-help group as an opportunity for 'exceptional desensitisation', self-disclosure of stammering and raising awareness of stammering in public speaking contexts.

They go on to discuss the key differences between self-help and therapy groups, including issues of access, leadership roles, contrasting aims, remits and processes. Possible roles a therapist could play (e.g. initiator, consultant, supporter) are described and how she might establish a new self-help group and/or maintain an existing one.

Membership of self-help groups are, without doubt, a crucial part of the long-term management of stammering. A clinician should view such an organisation as a vital resource and include supporting their work in her area of responsibility. The final word of this section is written by a group member and quoted by Liddle and Adams (2021):

"After months of angst, I finally plucked up the courage to go to a group meeting. To say I was anxious is an understatement; I felt physically sick. I'd planned in advance that I would only go to the first part of the meeting, but it was so brilliant that I decided to stay for the whole evening. I immediately felt at home. Everyone was so friendly and supportive. It was a major turning point in my life."

(p. 225)

REFERENCES

Beilby, J.M., Byrnes, M.L., Meagher, E.L. & Yaruss, J.S. (2013). The impact of stuttering on adults who stutter and their partners. *Journal of Fluency Disorders*, 38, 1, 14–29.

Boberg, E. & Kully, D. (1985). *Comprehensive Stuttering Program*. San Diego: College-Hill Press.

Boberg, J.M. & Boberg, E. (1990). The other side of the block: The stutterer's spouse. *Journal of Fluency Disorders*, 15, 61–75.

Boyle, M. (2013). Psychological characteristics and perceptions of stuttering of adults who stutter with and without support group experience. *Journal of Fluency Disorders*, 38, 4, 368–381.

Corcoran, J.A. & Stewart, M. (1998). Stories of stuttering. A qualitative analysis of interview narratives. *Journal of Fluency Disorders*, 23, 247–264.

Hughes, C.D. (2007). *An Investigation of Family Relationships for People Who Stutter*. Master's thesis, Bowling Green State University.

Hughes, S., Gabel, R., Irani, F. & Schlagheck, A. (2010). University students' perception of the life effects of stuttering. *Journal of Communication Disorders*, 43, 1, 45–60.

Klassen, T.R. & Kroll, R.M. (2005). Opinions on stuttering and its treatment: A follow-up survey and cross-cultural comparison. *Journal of Speech-Language Pathology & Audiology*, 29, 2, 73–82.

Liddle, H. & Adams, B. (2021). Working with self-help groups. In T. Stewart (ed.), *Stammering Resources for Adults and Children: Integrating Evidence into Clinical Practice*. London: Routledge, Taylor & Francis Group.

Linn, G.W. & Caruso, A.J. (1998). Perspectives on the effects of stuttering on the formation and maintenance of intimate relationships. *Journal of Rehabilitation*, 64, 3, 12–15.

Manning, W.H. (2001). *Clinical Decision Making in Fluency Disorders*, 2nd edition. Vancouver, Canada: Singular.

Plexico, L., Manning, W.H. & DiLollo, A. (2005). A phenom-enological understanding of successful stuttering management. *Journal of Fluency Disorders*, 30, 1–22.

Rolland, J.S. (1994). In sickness and in health: The impact of illness on couples' relationships. *Journal of Marital & Family Therapy*, 20, 327–347.

Turnbull, J. & Stewart, T. (2017). *The Dysfluency Resource Book*, 2nd edition. London: Routledge, Taylor & Francis Group.

FINAL THOUGHTS

99. WHAT DO I WISH I HAD KNOWN FROM THE START?

For this text, I have asked other clinicians what they wish they had known when they started working with individuals who stammer. Readers will have seen their comments scattered throughout the book. In this final section, I will include my own answers to this question:

I wish I had not tried to be the expert at the start. I wish I had not pretended to know, when clearly I lacked knowledge and experience.

I wish I had realised that I could ask the PWS when I didn't know what to say, didn't know what the answer was or which way to go in therapy. When I was able to collaborate with the PWS, seeing him as the expert on his stammering, the whole process seemed to proceed much better.

I wish I had listened more. I learnt so much by hearing the narrative of the PWS, understood more from his thoughts and emotions and benefited professionally and personally by being quiet, in the moment with him.

100. THE DANCE

Those who know me well will have some appreciation of how I love to dance; they will have discerned that I dance with passion, joy and freedom.

My work within the field of stammering has some similarities with my love of dance. I am passionate about stammering; I have a desire to know and understand stammering, principally from the perspective of those individuals who stammer. While writing this text, I have been struck by the surge in research

 DOI: 10.4324/9781003177890-13

exploring the PWS awareness of stammering. It is heartening to know that at last the PWS is coming to be recognised as a source of valuable knowledge and experience.

As a therapist, I have found a freedom to express an important vocation that I discovered I had at an early age. My understanding of various psychological approaches, especially the psychology of change, has enhanced my clinical skills and my own development in the field. I have found joy in being part of the journeys of numerous PWS. I am grateful to each of them for allowing me to play a role in their change processes.

And finally: My wishes. For those newly qualified therapists and those starting to specialise in the field of stammering, I have two wishes to gift to you:

I wish you the same freedom to express yourselves as I have felt.

I wish you joy in each and every clinical engagement.

APPENDIX 1: FORMAL ASSESSMENTS CURRENTLY IN USE

ACCEPTANCE

1. Acceptance and Action Questionnaire (AAQ-II) Bond, F.W., Hayes, S.C., Baer, R.A., Carpenter, K.M., Orcutt, H.K., Waltz, T. & Zettle, R.D. (2011). Preliminary psychometric properties of the acceptance and action questionnaire-II: A revised measure of psychological inflexibility and experiential avoidance. *Behavior Therapy*, 42, 676–688.

ANXIETY

1. Anxiety Inventory. Beck, A.T., Epstein, N., Brown, G. & Steer, R.A. (1988). An inventory for measuring clinical anxiety: Psychometric properties. *Journal of Consulting and Clinical Psychology*, 56, 893–897.
2. Multicomponent Anxiety Inventory e MCAI–IV. Schalling, D., Chronholm, B., Asberg, M. & Espmark, S. (1973). Ratings of psychic and somatic anxiety indicants: Interrater reliability and relations to personality variables. *Acta Psychiatrica Scandinavia*, 49, 353–368.
3. State-Trait Anxiety Inventory. Spielberger, C.D., Gorssuch, R.L., Lushene, P.R., Vagg, P.R. & Jacobs, G.A. (1983). *Manual for the State-Trait Anxiety Inventory*. Palo Alto, CA: Consulting Psychologists Press.
4. Social phobia and anxiety inventory. Turner, S.M., Beidel, D.C. & Dancu, C.V. (1996). *SPAI: Social Phobia and Anxiety Inventory Manual*. New York, NY: Multi-Health Systems Inc.
5. Social Phobia and Anxiety Inventory. Rodebaugh, T.L., Chambless, D.L., Terrill, D.R., Floyd, M. & Uhde, T. (2000).

Convergent, discriminant, and criterion-related validity of the Social Phobia and Anxiety Inventory. *Depression & Anxiety*, 11, 10–14.

DEPRESSION

1. Beck Depression Inventory. Beck, A.T., Steer, R.A. & Garbin, M.G. (1988). Psychometric properties of the Beck Depression Inventory: Twenty-five years of evaluation. *Clinical Psychology Review*, 8, 1, 77–100.
2. Beck Depression Inventory-II. Beck, A.T. (1996). *The Beck Depression Inventory-II*. San Antonio, TX: Psychological Corporation.

LOCUS OF CONTROL

1. Locus of Control Scale. Craig, A., Franklin, J. & Andrews, G. (1984). A scale to measure locus of control of behaviour. *British Journal of Medical Psychology*, 57, 173–180.

READINESS TO CHANGE

1. Readiness to change. McConnaughy, E.A., Prochaska, J.O. & Velicer, W.F. (1983). Stages of change in psychotherapy: Measurement and sample profiles. *Psychotherapy: Theory, Research & Practice*, 20, 368–375.

SEVERITY RATING

1. SSI-4. Riley, G.D. (2009). *Stuttering Severity Instrument for Children and Adults (SSI-4)*, 4th edition. Austin, TX: Pro-Ed, Inc.
2. S24 scale. Andrews, G. & Cutler, J. (1974). S-24 Scale – Stuttering therapy: The relations between changes in symptom level and attitudes. *Journal of Speech & Hearing Disorders*, 39, 312–319.

SPEAKERS' EXPERIENCE OF STAMMERING

1. Perceptions of Stuttering Inventory. Woolf, G. (1967). The assessment of stuttering as struggle, avoidance and

expectancy. *British Journal of Disorders Communication,* 2, 158–171.

2. Stuttering Self-Rating Profile (WASSP) Wright, L. & Ayre, A. (2000). *Stuttering Self-Rating Profile.* Bicester, UK: Winslow Press.

3. (OASES) Yaruss, J.S. & Quesal, R.W. (2006). Overall assessment of the speaker's experience of stuttering: Documenting multiple outcomes in stuttering treatment. *Journal of Fluency Disorders,* 31, 90–115.

4. Satisfaction with Communication in Everyday Speaking Situations scale. Karimi, H., Onslow, M., Jones, M., O'Brian, S., Packman, A., Menzies, R., Reilly, S., Sommer, M. & Jelcic-Jaksic, S. (2018). The Satisfaction with Communication in Everyday Speaking Situations (SCESS) scale: An overarching outcome measure of treatment effect. *Journal of Fluency Disorders,* 58, 77–85.

THOUGHTS/COGNITIONS

1. Fear of Negative Evaluation Scale. Leary, M.R. (1983). A brief version of the Fear of Negative Evaluation Scale. *Personality & Social Psychology Bulletin,* 9, 371–375.

2. Social Avoidance and Distress and Fear of Negative Evaluation Scales. Turner, S.M., McCanna, M. & Beidel, D.C. (1987). Validity of the Social Avoidance and Distress and Fear of Negative Evaluation Scales. *Behaviour Research & Therapy,* 25, 113–115.

3. Unhelpful Thoughts and Beliefs About Stuttering. St Clare, T., Menzies, R., Onslow, M., Packman, A., Thompson, R. & Block, S. (2009). Unhelpful thoughts and beliefs linked to social anxiety in stuttering: Development of a measure. *International Journal of Language and Communication Disorders,* 44, 3, 338–351.

   A Brief Version of the Unhelpful Thoughts and Beliefs about Stuttering Scales: The UTBAS-6. Iverach, L., Heard, R., Menzies, R., Lowe, R., O'Brian, S., Packman, A. & Onslow, M. (2016). *Journal of Speech, Language, & Hearing Research,* 59, 5, 964–972.

OTHER

1. Stuttering Assessment. Crowe, T.A., Di Lollo, A. & Crowe, B.T. (2000). *Crowe's Protocols: A Comprehensive Guide to Stuttering Assessment.* San Antonio, TX: The Psychological Corporation.
2. Psychological Assessment. Groth-Marnat, G. (1990). *The Handbook of Psychological Assessment,* 2nd edition. New York: John Wiley & Sons.

100 NAVIGATIONAL POINTS: DYSFLUENCY

APPENDIX 2: COGNITIVE RESTRUCTURING: LEARNING TO MANAGE UNHELPFUL THOUGHTS

Unhelpful thought.

_____

1. What evidence do you have for the thought?

_____
_____
_____

2. What evidence do you have against the thought?

_____
_____
_____

3. What would you tell a friend (to help them) if they had the thought?

_____
_____
_____

4. Think of your calmest, most rational and supportive friend or family member. How would he/she react to the causal thought? What would he/she say?

_____
_____
_____

5. Are you worrying about an outcome you can't control? Is there any point to this type of worry?

_____
_____
_____

6. What does the thought do for you? How does it make you feel? Is it helpful in any way, or is it just distressing?

_____

_____

_____

7. What good things would you gain if you gave up the thought? How would your life be different if you didn't believe the thought?

_____

_____

_____

8. If the causal thought were true, what is the worst outcome? Is it as bad as you think?

_____

_____

_____

(Menzies et al. 2009)

STATEMENTS IN THE UNHELPFUL THOUGHTS AND BELIEFS ABOUT STUTTERING (UTBAS) SCALE (ST CLARE ET AL. 2009)

1. People will doubt my ability because I stutter
2. It's impossible to be really successful in life if you stutter
3. I won't be able to keep a job if I stutter
4. It's all my fault – I should be able to control my stutter
5. I'm a weak person because I stutter
6. No one will like me if I stutter
7. I might stutter
8. People focus on every word I say
9. I am incompetent
10. No one could love a stutterer
11. I will stutter
12. Everyone in the room will hear me stutter
13. I'm stupid
14. Other people will think I'm stupid if I stutter
15. I'll never be successful because of my stutter

16. I won't be able to answer their questions
17. I'm hopeless
18. I'm of no use in the workplace
19. People will think I'm incompetent because I stutter
20. I'll block completely and won't be able to talk
21. Everyone will think I'm an idiot
22. I can't speak to people in positions of authority
23. People will think I'm strange
24. People will think I can't speak English
25. No one would want to have a relationship with a stutterer
26. I can't think clearly because I stutter
27. I can't speak to aggressive people
28. People will think that I have no opinions
29. People will think I'm boring because I have nothing to say
30. If I block, people will think I'm retarded
31. I can't face these people
32. People will wonder what's wrong with me if I stutter
33. What will people think of me if they disagree with what I say?
34. Most people view stutterers as less capable
35. I don't want to go – people won't like me
36. My pauses are too long – people will think I'm weird
37. People won't like me because I won't be able to talk
38. I can't convince people of anything I say because I stutter
39. People will think I'm retarded if I stutter
40. I'll block – I know I will
41. I'll make a fool of myself
42. People get tired of waiting for me to get my words out
43. People shouldn't have to wait so long for me to speak
44. I always embarrass the people I'm speaking to
45. People think I have something to hide because my stutter sounds suspicious
46. People will think that I'm worthless
47. I'll embarrass myself
48. I can't speak to people I find sexually attractive
49. No one will understand what I'm trying to say
50. What's the point of even trying to speak – it never comes out right

51. I won't be able to say exactly what I want to say
52. Everyone will think I'm simple or dumb because I avoid using difficult words
53. I slow up everyone's conversation
54. Everyone hates it when I start to speak
55. I can never speak on the phone
56. I won't be able to ask for what I want
57. The person on the other end of the phone will hang up on me
58. People will laugh at me
59. People will think I'm mute
60. I'll never finish explaining my point – they'll misunderstand me
61. The answering machine will turn off if I block – I won't be able to leave any message
62. They'll think I'm a prank caller if I block
63. I won't be able to say 'hello' when I pick up the phone
64. People who stutter are stupid
65. People who stutter are incompetent
66. People who stutter are boring

INDEX

Page numbers in *italics* indicate a figure and page numbers in **bold** indicate a table on the corresponding page.

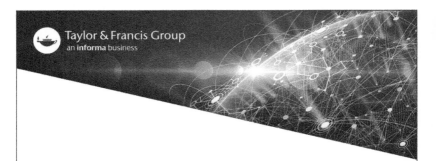

For Product Safety Concerns and Information please contact our EU
representative GPSR@taylorandfrancis.com Taylor & Francis Verlag GmbH,
Kaufingerstraße 24, 80331 München, Germany

Printed and bound by CPI Group (UK) Ltd, Croydon, CR0 4YY
08/06/2025
01896991-0001